THE DELVIN REPORT ON SAFER SEX

The Delvin Report On Safer Sex is for the
millions of people who *enjoy* sex and want to
go on enjoying it.
Clearly set out are the descriptions of what's
safe and what's to be avoided, advice on
assessing your own risks and how to lessen
them. It also gives the full medical facts about
AIDS and all the other sexually transmitted
diseases, about contraception methods and
safety precautions.
The Delvin Report On Safer Sex shows that
these can still be the Enjoyable Eighties.

About the author

Dr. David Delvin is Consultant Editor of
General Practitioner and Medical Consultant
to the Family Planning Association. He has
appeared in hundreds of radio and television
programmes, and has been Medical Adviser
to such TV programmes as *Pebble Mill at
One*, *Medical Express*, *Inside Medicine*, *The
Afternoon Programme*, *Aspel and Company*,
and *About Anglia*.
He writes regular columns for national
magazines and for various medical journals.
His books, which include THE BOOK OF LOVE,
HOW TO IMPROVE YOUR SEX LIFE,
CAREFREE LOVE and TAKING THE PILL, have
been translated into eight languages and one
has won the Best Book Award of The
American Medical Writers' Association. He
recently won the 'Consumer Columnist of the
Year' award, and was awarded the *Médaille
de la Ville de Paris* by Jacques Chirac.

The Delvin Report on Safer Sex
(in the AIDS era)

Dr David Delvin

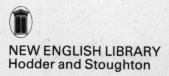
NEW ENGLISH LIBRARY
Hodder and Stoughton

First published in Great Britain in
1988 by New English Library
Paperbacks

British Library C.I.P.

Delvin, David
  The Delvin report on safer sex:
(in the AIDS era).
  1. Sexual intercourse
  I. Title
613.9′6   HQ31

ISBN 0 450 41907 X

Printed and bound in Great Britain
for Hodder and Stoughton
Paperbacks, a division of Hodder
and Stoughton Ltd., Mill Road,
Dunton Green, Sevenoaks, Kent
TN13 2YA. (Editorial Office:
47 Bedford Square, London
WC1B 3DP) by Richard Clay Ltd.,
Bungay, Suffolk. Photoset by
Rowland Phototypesetting Ltd.,
Bury St Edmunds, Suffolk.

To C.C.W., with love

Acknowledgements

My thanks to Valerie Woods for her typing; to Christina Roe for her last-minute help; to Quantime Computer Company, Fiona Moody and Catherine Whitehead for processing the figures; and to the Post Office – for not losing the manuscript for very long.

Thanks also to SHE magazine (and to Joyce Hopkirk, Eric Bailey and Hilary Smith) for commissioning and backing the survey.

CONTENTS

CHAPTER NINE:
Achieving Your Orgasm – And Achieving It Safely

What the Delvin Report revealed about orgasms ● Why you shouldn't let the search for orgasms dominate your sex life ● Secrets of easily orgasmic women ● What makes them "easy comers"? ● How they first reached orgasm ● What was first intercourse like for them? ● Are these women's sexual partners something special? ● How they use fantasy in bed to reach a climax ● The importance of communication ● Where do they like being touched? ● Clitoral pleasure

CHAPTER TEN:
Safe (But Sexy) Ways To Use Contraception – Including How To Cope With Condoms

Which methods are most popular today? ● The condom: an up-and-coming method of safe sex ● The cap or diaphragm ● The sponge ● The Pill ● The Mini-Pill ● The IUD (loop, coil) and infection ● Spermicides and their alleged anti-AIDS activity ● Rhythm method (and its variations) ● Vasectomy ● Female sterilisation ● The Shot ● Effectiveness of the various methods ● A warning about abortion

CHAPTER ELEVEN:
Sex In The Nervous Nineties – And The Way Male/Female Relationships Are Changing

How sex is changing ● The effects of the AIDS panic ● The puritan backlash ● Male/female relationships ● What will women expect of men in the 1990s? ● Safe sex

FURTHER READING

INTRODUCTION

Why You Need This Book

If you've ever had sex, you need to read this book. In fact, even if you've *never* had sex, but think you might do one day, you'd better read it!

Why?

Because the whole sexual ball-game (if you'll forgive the phrase) has changed dramatically in the last few years.

Very, very alarming things are happening – things which make a night's fun in bed much riskier than it was before. Things like this:

★ *AIDS* is increasing at a terrifying rate, and is now hitting ordinary "straight" (i.e. heterosexual) people as well as the male gays who were the first to be struck down so tragically by it.

★ *Herpes* is making those agreeable romantic affairs decidedly risky – and indeed a trifle like Russian roulette in many parts of the world!

★ *Cancer of the cervix* is affecting large numbers of women: particularly (I'm afraid) those who've had multiple, and perhaps badly-chosen, sexual partners – but also those who've always been faithful to one man.

★ *Infertility* is affecting many women – because their tubes have been blocked by unnoticed infections picked up during past sexual frolics.

But despite all that gloom, I hope to show you in this book that sex is STILL great fun, and that *if you play things sensibly*, you can still have a wonderful time in bed.

Whether you're single, married or divorced (or even – dare I say it – *widowed*: for a surprising proportion of my "agony uncle" postbag is from merry widows and widowers who still lead active sex lives), it's worth bearing in mind that love-making is still one of the greatest of all gifts to humanity.

Yes, despite all the fears about AIDS, herpes, cancer and VD, it remains true that sex – preferably with someone you really love – remains a source of immense pleasure, comfort, tenderness and reassurance to tens of millions of people all over the world.

And I'm not exaggerating when I say "tens of millions"; did you know that a recent estimate says that at any given instant in time, no less than *7¾ million* people are making love to each other? No wonder there are so many babies in the world!

Love-making is something so beautiful and so satisfying to the human emotions that it helps countless people make some sense of a difficult, risky and uncertain world.

This book will – I hope – assist *you* to enjoy the thrills and fulfilment of love-making without unnecessary fear of the "new dangers", like AIDS and cervical cancer. And if you love somebody, I hope it'll help you to strengthen that relationship and to have a marvellous time in bed together – without having to worry about unpleasant consequences.

The book will also tell you one very important thing: *which sex practices are safe, and which AREN'T*.

My recent Delvin Report sex survey of 6,000 British women revealed that large numbers of them are doing things in bed which are downright dangerous to their health! In the middle chapters of this book, I'm going to describe those practices and tell you *why* they're so dodgy.

On the positive side, the Delvin Report revealed that a lot of couples are finding new, exciting, inventive and thoroughly *safe* things to do in the bedroom. (No, NOT swinging from the chandelier, sir – the flex might break and leave you impaled on the bedpost. . . .)

So I'll also be describing these safe – and highly agreeable – bedtime activities.

Read on – and have a great time!

Dr. David Delvin

CHAPTER ONE

Sex Is Still Fun – But How Much At Risk Are You?

Don't be too scared by panic headlines ● What's AIDS anyway? ● What's herpes? ● What's cancer of the cervix? ● Why have all these troubles hit us? ● From the "Swinging Sixties" to the "Nervous Nineties" : Lucy's case history ● Claire's case history ● The importance of assessing your own risk ● An AIDS risk quiz for women ● An AIDS risk quiz for men

Don't be too scared by panic headlines

There are going to be some pretty scary headlines about sex in the next few years – scary enough to put many a man or woman off it altogether!

I'm not joking: we're already beginning to see patients who've developed severe emotional and sexual "hang-ups" because they've got so frightened about AIDS, herpes and cancer.

But there's really no need for all that. As this book will show you, the average heterosexual person who's *sensible* about his or her love-life (and who obtains commonsense health checks where necessary) is at very low risk of running into danger from any of these diseases.

Note the word "heterosexual": I'm afraid that I can't offer the same comfort to gay blokes – who really are going to be in terrible danger from AIDS during the next few years.

(*Female* gays, by the way, are NOT at any special risk; in fact they run into less health problems in the genital area than we heterosexuals do. This is mainly due to the gentle and non-penetrative nature of their love play.)

But to be frank, this book *isn't* for gay people, who must seek help and advice elsewhere – for instance, from hard-working organisations like the Terrence Higgins Trust (01-833 2971).

No, this book is basically for "straight" people: ideally, a loving couple should read it together and see what the risks of sex are for both of them – and find out how they can minimise these risks.

So don't panic when you see daft headlines saying:

★"EPIDEMIC OF CERVICAL CANCER" (it's quite common, but there certainly isn't an epidemic).
★"ONE MILLION CASES OF HERPES IN ENGLAND" (there were only 20,000 last year).
★"WILL AIDS WIPE OUT BRITAIN?" (No, it won't.)

Well, out of the three dangers listed in those headlines, the one that's causing the most alarm and despondency at the moment is AIDS.

So let's begin having a brief look at what AIDS is. I'll be explaining the disease in much more detail in Chapter Seven, but here's a brief outline of a much-misunderstood infection.

What's AIDS anyway?

AIDS is an always-fatal illness, caused by a virus.

The virus is not killed by any antibiotic – and I must be blunt and say that at the moment it seems to me that there's absolutely *no* prospect of any drug being found in the next few years that will cure the disease.

It *may* be possible to find a vaccine which would stop

people catching the virus – and one is on trial now. But that'll be no help to those who've already got it.

The virus is called "HIV". The most "efficient" ways of passing it on are:

★Rectal sex (which is why it has hit male gays so badly);
★Transfusion of infected blood (now very, very rare in most Western countries);
★Injection of other blood products (such as the special blood factor which is needed by haemophiliac children and adults);
★Using "shared" needles (which is why the virus spreads like wildfire among users of injectable drugs).

There's more about rarer ways of catching AIDS in Chapter Seven. But for the moment, I just want to make two points about transmission of HIV virus:

★You don't catch it by ordinary social contact;
★Unfortunately, you CAN catch it through "straight" man–woman vaginal sex.

It's not as easy to catch it through vaginal intercourse as it is through rectal intercourse. Quite a few people have vaginal sex with an infected partner and get away with it – and the reasons *why* they get away with it still aren't clear. A condom gives you some protection – but it's not likely to be 100% safe.

If you catch the virus, you won't necessarily get AIDS. In the early days (that is, the early to middle 1980s), experts were cheerfully saying that only a small minority of people with the virus would develop AIDS.

That forecast now seems *very* over-optimistic. It now appears possible that most people who catch the HIV virus may eventually develop AIDS.

If you *do* develop the disease, what happens is this. The germ makes your body's defences against infection give up the ghost.

Therefore, you become a sitting duck for any infection

that comes along – particularly chest infections – and these infections may kill you.

In addition, the virus has the odd effect of causing a skin cancer called "Kaposi's sarcoma".

Finally, the HIV virus often attacks the brain, causing a severe dementia (that is, loss of intellect).

I haven't minced words in telling you that this is a truly terrible germ, which is going to kill very large numbers of the population over the next few years.

I think you can see that the only real hope of defeating it (unless a vaccine suitable for mass use comes along) is for all of us to behave a heck of a lot more sensibly than we did in the years of the Permissive Society.

This book will tell you how.

What's herpes?

Herpes was *the* big sexual scare story before AIDS. Of course, AIDS has now pushed it out of the headlines – but it's still increasing, and still causing a great deal of pain, distress and ill-health (as well as ruining a lot of people's sex lives).

What is it? It's an infection of the sex organs – again caused by a virus.

This one is very similar to the one which causes "cold sores" on people's lips.

It's passed on by sexual contact, and it produces painful little blisters on the sex organs.

That may not sound too bad. But if I tell you that herpes can cause really *intense* pain in some people, and that it can lead to serious urinary problems, and that it may possibly be a cause of cancer of the cervix (see below), you'll see that it's no joke.

Add to that the fact that it tends to keep coming back year after year – and also the fact that there's no drug that will cure it. You can see that it's a pretty nasty thing to have.

I'll explain herpes more fully in Chapter Eight. But meantime, if you bear in mind that it can be passed on by just a few moments of sexual intercourse with an infected person, you'll see that by far the most effective way of preventing it is to avoid potentially risky sexual liaisons.

What's cancer of the cervix?

You can see where the cervix is from Figure 1.

Also known as the "neck of the womb", it's the little soft lump which can be felt at the top end of a woman's vagina.

Figure 1 also shows what happens during intercourse: the man's penis bangs repeatedly against the cervix. It's thought that this repeated slight trauma is one of the causes of cancer of the cervix.

Why? Heaven knows! But possibly intercourse may introduce a virus – carried by the man on his penis – into the delicate tissues of the cervix.

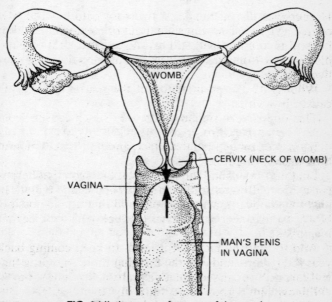

FIG. 1 Likely cause of cancer of the cervix.

Certainly, it appears to be a fact that the more lovers a woman has had, the more likely she is to get cancer of the cervix, I'm afraid.

Symptoms and prevention of this very serious (but avoidable) disorder are discussed in Chapter Eight. And whether you're a man or a woman, one obvious thing you can do to help prevent the spread of this disease is to follow the "safe sex" rules given in this book.

Why have all these troubles hit us?

I'm afraid that there's only one reason why all these sexual troubles have hit the world – permissiveness.

I'm not playing the heavy moralist in saying this! I just think it's a medical fact. The sexual permissiveness of the 1960s, 1970s and 1980s has (let's face it) been enormously agreeable for many people.

There's really no point in denying that, for the first time in history, very large numbers of men and women have been able to go to bed with a wide range of partners and have a great time – with little risk of social disgrace or unwanted pregnancy.

But alas, there were other risks which most of us hadn't reckoned with – particularly the risk of germs (such as the viruses of AIDS and herpes).

You see, germs have an astonishing ability to exploit any new form of human behaviour, and to use it to their own advantage.

Let me give you an example. Until recent years, very few parents sent their pre-school kids to nursery school or playschool. So, youngsters under the age of six weren't often exposed to respiratory germs – and as a result, respiratory infections were quite uncommon in the 2–5 age group.

Today, playschools have mushroomed all over the place. Very nice: but one consequence has been the fact that large numbers of toddlers now go down with respiratory viruses – because they're being exposed to so many of them through fairly close nose and mouth contact with other kids and teachers!

In the same way, the extraordinary explosion of sexual contact during the period 1960 to the present day has caused a fantastic increase in the incidence of certain infections which were previously very rare, or confined to very small geographical areas of the world.

The most extreme example of a change in human sexual behaviour leading to an epidemic is of course the terrible AIDS outbreak among gay men. Thirty years ago, homosexuality was forbidden by law (and subject to very harsh penalties) in Britain and most Western countries.

In the 60s, laws were generally relaxed and gays were able to be much more open. Gay sex contacts became much commoner. Unfortunately, some people took this to extremes: in gay "bath-houses" in certain cities, it was possible for a man to go in the door at 10p.m. and to come out again at midnight – having had some sort of sexual contact with fifty different blokes!

I'm afraid the AIDS virus must have thought this sudden change was Christmas and birthday rolled into one.

So without being condemnatory of anyone, I think it's quite obvious that the only way for us to defeat these diseases is to modify our sexual behaviour so that there's less chance of passing these germs on.

If we don't do so, then I would confidently forecast that NEW sexually-transmitted germs will emerge by the 1990s to trouble the poor old human race. (There are already rumours of unpleasant new variants of HIV, I'm afraid.)

From the "Swinging Sixties" to the "Nervous Nineties": Lucy's case history

To illustrate the point I've been making, let me tell you about the case history of Lucy – a typical "child of the 60s".

Back in 1962, Lucy was 22, a fashion model and a virgin. (Yes, virginity at 22 was common in those days!)

Then very suddenly indeed, along came the much freer

attitudes to love-making which seemed to go with Beatles music, pot-smoking and flower-power.

Lucy decided to sleep with the boy friend who she'd been doing nothing but heavy petting with for two years (such relatively chaste arrangements were quite the norm in 1962!).

She liked the experience of intercourse, and soon decided that she ought to try it out with some other boys. By 1966, she had a successful career – and a track record of twenty-seven lovers.

Thanks to the Pill (use of which became widespread in the late 60s) she avoided unwanted pregnancy – though she did have a series of troublesome vaginal infections in the 1970s.

By 1975, she was attending show business "orgy-parties", partly in the hope of getting work. At some of these, she'd have sex with a dozen men, and perhaps one or two women as well.

In 1980, she decided to settle down and get married: there was still just time for her to have a child, which she very much wanted.

By the mid-1980s, it was clear that she was *never* going to have a baby. The reason? Her tubes were "shot to pieces" with pelvic inflammatory disease: P.I.D. (please see Chapter Eight) – the chronic infection which has made so many "children of the 60s" into the infertile would-be mothers of the 80s. In her case, it was caused by gonorrhoea – which had produced no symptoms and therefore gone undiagnosed.

Meanwhile, Lucy's husband is cheerfully playing around with other women, and having "a girl on the side" most weeks. As we move into the "Nervous Nineties", there's little doubt as to what Lucy will be worrying about over the next few years: will he bring home AIDS?

Claire's case history

Lucy, you must admit, was a bit of a little raver, to put it mildly!

Far more typical of women today is somebody like Claire.

She's a suburban housewife, married with three children. She had a couple of lovers back in the 60s before she got married. And after her third child was born, she had a brief, passionate, and now much-regretted affair with her brother-in-law.

Claire wrote to me at one of my advice columns, because she had become terrified that God would punish her for her past, and give her cancer of the cervix or AIDS.

In fact, her risk of cancer of the cervix is pretty low – *provided* she has regular smear tests. And her risk of having acquired AIDS from her past frolics is just about nil, unless her brother-in-law has gay tendencies or (wildly unlikely) is a haemophiliac.

The importance of assessing your own risk

Like most of the people who write to me about AIDS, Claire had totally misjudged her own level of risk, which was really very small. (Lucy's would be much higher – at least, if her husband keeps "screwing around".)

I'm deluged with letters from people who think they're in great danger of AIDS when they aren't – and I also get letters from people who smugly reckon that they're in no danger of it, when in fact they're prime targets for the virus.

So I feel that it's very important for you to *assess your own risk carefully*.

When you've done that, you can decide whether your sex life needs adjusting in any way.

To help you, I've put together a short "Are you at risk?" questionnaire, with separate sections for men and women. It'll only take you a few minutes to complete, and it'll tell you whether you're high or low risk.

N.B. Do bear in mind that even "Low Risk" people can get AIDS – so don't do anything silly!

Here goes:

An AIDS risk quiz for women

1. Since 1980, have you had a blood transfusion *outside Europe*?

   Yes (50 points) No (0 points)

2. Since 1980, have you used any injectable drugs?

   Yes (250 points) No (0 points)

3. Have you used any in the last year?

   Yes (600 points) No (0 points)

4. Are you a virgin?

   Yes (0 points – and go directly to the assessment at the end of the quiz. Do not collect £200.) No (50 points)

5. Roughly how many men have you slept with since 1980?

   Count 5 points for each one.

6. And how many men have you slept with in the last year?

   Count an *extra* 10 points for each of these.

7. Would you describe any of your partners during the last year as very promiscuous?

   Yes (100 points) No (0 points)

8. As far as you know, have any of the partners of the last twelve months been on injectable drugs (at any time)?

   Yes (500 points for each one) No (0 points)

9. Would you describe any of them as bisexual?

   Yes (400 points for each one) No (0 points)

10.	Had any of them visited Central or West Africa on tourism or business recently (i.e. in the year before you made love with them)?	Yes (50 points for each one)	No (0 points)
11.	Had any of them visited New York or San Francisco in the previous year?	Yes (20 points for each one)	No (0 points)
12.	Are any of them haemophiliac?	Yes (600 points)	No (0 points)
13.	Have *you* been to Central or West Africa or to New York or San Francisco in the last year?	Yes (50 points)	No (0 points)
14.	Did you have sex with anybody who was living there?	Yes (50 points)	No (0 points)
15.	Have you been abroad anywhere else on a business trip by yourself, or on a "singles holiday" in the last year?	Yes (20 points)	No (0 points)
16.	Has your current boy friend or husband been abroad without you in the last year?	Yes (40 points)	No (0 points)
17.	Forgive the question, but have you gone in for rectal sex in the last year – and if so, with how many men?	Yes (20 points for each man)	No (0 points)
18.	When you make love, does your partner wear a condom?	Always (0 points) Sometimes (30 points) Never (60 points)	

Assessment for women

If you scored 0–65 points: You are at no risk at all from AIDS.

If you scored 70–350 points: Your risk of AIDS is at present terribly low – and probably not worth worrying about. But if you're at the top end of the range, there are bound to be one or two obvious aspects of your past life-style which could put you at slight risk.

If you scored 355–550 points: You seem to be at slightly higher than average risk for a woman. Look at your life-style, and your recent partners, and see what action needs to be taken. More detailed advice in Chapter Seven.

If you scored 555–1000 points: Your recent lifestyle – and probably your choice of partners – is clearly putting you at some considerable risk. You should *definitely* alter the way you're living and stop having sex with risky partners. It may be worth seeing a counsellor and discussing the possibility of a blood test for AIDS virus.

If you scored over 1000 points: I'm afraid you could be in big trouble very soon. You certainly need a blood test NOW, and you should go to a Genito-Urinary ("Special") Clinic and see the counsellor there.

An AIDS risk quiz for men

1.	Are you basically gay?	Yes (100 points – and go directly to Question 25)	No (0 points)
2.	Are you bisexual?	Yes (100 points – and go directly to Question 25)	No (0 points)

3. Since 1980, have you had a blood transfusion *outside* Europe?
Yes (50 points) No (0 points)

4. Since 1980, have you used any injectable drugs?
Yes (250 points) No (0 points)

5. Have you used any in the last year?
Yes (600 points) No (0 points)

6. Are you haemophiliac?
Yes (700 points) No (0 points)

7. Have you ever made love to a woman?
Yes (50 points) No (0 points – and go directly to the assessment at the end of the quiz.)

8. Roughly how many women have you slept with since 1985?
Count 5 points for each one.

9. And how many have you slept with in the last year?
Count 10 points for each one.

10. Would you describe any of these women during the last year as being very promiscuous?
Yes (100 points) No (0 points)

11. As far as you know, have any of your partners of the last year been on injectable drugs at any time?
Yes (500 points) No (0 points)

12. Did any of them visit New York or San Francisco on tourism or business the year before you slept with them?
Yes (20 points) No (0 points)

		Yes	No
13.	Had any of them visited Central or West Africa in the previous year?	Yes (50 points)	No (0 points)
14.	Have any of them told you that they'd recently (i.e. in the previous year) had a bisexual boy friend?	Yes (400 points)	No (0 points)
15.	Have you yourself been to Central or West Africa in the last year?	Yes (50 points)	No (0 points)
16.	If "Yes", then did you have sex with anybody there?	Yes (200 points)	No (0 points)
17.	And if the answer to Question 16 was "Yes", was she a prostitute?	Yes (500 points)	No (0 points)
18.	Have you been to New York or San Francisco in the last year?	Yes (50 points)	No (0 points)
19.	If "Yes", did you have sex with anybody there?	Yes (100 points)	No (0 points)
20.	If the answer was "Yes", was she a prostitute?	Yes (200 points)	No (0 points)
21.	Have you been abroad on a "singles holiday" or solo business trip in the last year?	Yes (40 points)	No (0 points)
22.	Has your current girl friend or wife been abroad without you in the last year?	Yes (40 points)	No (0 points)

14

23. Have you had rectal sex with anyone in the last year?	Yes (15 points)	No (0 points)
24. When you make love, do you wear a condom?	Always (0 points) Sometimes (30 points) Never (60 points)	
25. For gay and bisexual men only: how many male partners have you had in the last year?	Count 200 points for each one.	
26. Also for gay and bisexual males: do you engage in passive – i.e. receptive – anal sex? (*Note:* it would obviously be possible to do a far more in-depth profile for gay/bisexual males, but this book is primarily intended for heterosexual men and women.)	Yes (200 points)	No (0 points)

Assessment for men

If you scored 0–65 points: You're at practically no risk at all from AIDS. In fact, you may as well take this book back to the library or bookshop!

If you scored 70–350 points: At present, your risk is very low – but watch your life-style in the future, especially if you tend to sleep around.

If you scored 355–550 points: Slightly higher than average risk. Take care!

If you scored 555–1000 points: You're at considerably greater than average risk. Think about modifying your behaviour now. If you're at the high end of the range, consider going to see an AIDS counsellor (see below).

If you scored over 1000 points: I'm afraid you're definitely in the "High Risk" group. It's time to see a counsellor at your local STD ("Special") Clinic and – if he/she agrees – have a blood test.

CHAPTER TWO

Sex In Britain Today – The Findings Of "The Delvin Report"

*Why it's important to know what people are doing in bed ●
The Delvin Report and what it reveals about late 1980s
women ● The orgasmic, liberated ladies of Britain ● The
more saddening results of the survey ● A cheerful picture of
late 1980s sex life ● Hearing about the "facts of life" ● First
menstruation ● First sexual feelings ● First kissing, and first
petting ● First intercourse ● First orgasm ● Masturbation ●
How women rate their sex lives today ● How many times per
week? ● How many orgasms per week? ● More orgasmic
questions ● Adultery ● Women's relationship with men ●
Rape and child abuse ● Changing sexual behaviour ● Sex
between women*

Why it's important to know what people are doing in bed

There's a great deal of muddle and mis-information about
what people actually get up to in bed.

Indeed, I find that most men and women are surprised to
find that anyone does anything different from what *they* do
in the bedroom!

So I reckon there's a definite need for an occasional sex
survey to keep us all up to date about what people are
actually doing in between the sheets.

That's particularly important at the present time when it

17

seems likely that many people's sexual behaviour is starting to change as a result of the AIDS threat.

The Delvin Report and what it reveals about late 1980s women

Hence the Delvin Report – which I recently conducted with the help of *She*, the popular British monthly magazine for women.

We published a frank, open questionnaire containing a large number of *very* blunt queries about readers' sex lives – and whether they were proposing to change them in view of AIDS and other dangers.

Eventually, I received some 6,000 replies from women who were kind enough to help us. Although all the respondents were female, what they told me does reveal a very great deal about *men's* sex lives too!

I'd like to express my sincere thanks to everyone who took the trouble to fill in a form and return it to me. Now the final results have been collated, we have a piece of sexological research of considerable importance, which gives a remarkable insight into the love-lives of women of all ages in all parts of the British Isles.

But perhaps more importantly, a lot of women who responded to the survey very kindly took the trouble to add notes, or even long letters, saying that filling in the questionnaire had helped them to sort out their sex lives quite a bit.

One lady wrote: "It wasn't till I'd filled in the answers on your form that I realised what a rotter my man is. So I've dumped him – the pig!"

Another wrote: "I've been very muddled about my sexuality. But the experience of writing down what I actually feel about going to bed with men, and the reasons why I do it, has clarified my mind and helped me to think straight about sex for the first time. Many thanks."

Of course, the rather startling frankness of our survey questions didn't please everybody. Several questionnaires

18

were returned to me blank, but with decidedly shirty letters attached to them.

One of these read: "I am not filling in this form, because it mentions practices which can lead to AIDS. Didn't you know that?"

Well, we did. And in fact, a major object of the survey was to discover whether women are changing their sexual behaviour as a result of the new fears of AIDS and herpes – and also whether they realise that certain common sex practices can be quite dangerous.

Another woman, who was clearly very sincere in her views, wrote: "I am never buying *She* again. I realise that some people might disagree with me, but they are *all perverted.*"

Well, I suppose you can't please everybody! I respect the views of the tiny handful of people who wrote in to protest about the sexually explicit nature of the survey. But I'm glad that it helped some people, and that most women clearly found it fun.

Indeed, many replies were splendidly witty, and confirmed my lifelong belief that the most important thing a woman can take to bed with her is a sense of humour!

However, there were some very sad replies too. It's quite clear from the survey that in the latter part of the 80s there are still many British women who are leading appallingly frustrating sex lives, or who are putting up with the kind of bedtime misery that should have gone out in Victorian days.

In particular, it seems that the "New Man" – so gallantly promoted by writers such as agony uncle and broadcaster Phillip Hodson – is nowhere near as common in late 1980s Britain as he should be. Many women are still going to bed with guys who are nothing more than old-style male chauvinist pigs!

A classic example was the first completed questionnaire which I picked up off the top of the pile, completely at random. In answer to the question, "Do you talk with your partner during love-play and love-making?" this reader

19

had replied: "I wish we could. But he doesn't allow me to speak in bed, because he says it puts him off."

"Allow" indeed! What a terrible indictment of a male –female relationship. And that questionnaire was only one of hundreds which had quite clearly been filled in by women who were still taking an all-too-submissive attitude to bossy and selfish husbands or lovers (or, in some cases, both . . .).

The orgasmic, liberated ladies of Britain

But looking on the brighter side, there's no doubt that most of the thousands of women who responded to the survey really are liberated and don't let men boss them around at bedtime.

They're interested in their own sexual satisfaction, as well as the man's. And the results show that in most cases, they certainly are getting it.

Indeed, among the most startling results of this survey are the very high frequencies of both intercourse and orgasm reported by a large number of the women who took part – in comparison to earlier sex surveys, such as Dr. Kinsey's of the early 1950s.

Some of the completed questionnaires reported so many lovers, so many episodes of intercourse a week, and so many orgams (whether through intercourse, through love play or through masturbation) that I must admit I don't entirely understand how the women in question find time for anything else in their lives.

Particularly striking was the high incidence of masturbation. Now, masturbation is something that traditionally women don't like to admit to, or indeed talk about. Even in the confidential atmosphere of a doctor's consulting room, this is one subject that is rarely broached.

Yet the figures do reveal that a quite staggering proportion of British women do regularly use a spot of "do-it-yourself" to bring themselves to a climax, or to relieve sexual frustration.

My study of the letters which accompanied so many questionnaires indicates that lots of women were actually pretty relieved to be able to put down on paper the "confession" that they regularly do something which they'd not really talked to anyone about before.

However, the letters also indicate that not *all* of these women are "solitary" masturbators. Many appear to do this to themselves after intercourse, as a way of ensuring that they reach a climax, sometimes after the bloke has fallen asleep. (Gentlemen – did you *realise* that this was what was going on while you were snoring away?)

So, with or without a partner, the late 1980s woman appears – judged by the standards of previous surveys in this field – to be having more sexual enjoyment than ever before. Indeed, much of this survey is, thank heavens, a sheer celebration of sexual joy – and of the happiness of being a sexually active woman in a world that no longer denies a female the right to enjoy the sensuality of her own body.

The more saddening results of the survey

But there are some saddening results too. My staff who first reviewed the summary of the computer print-out were amazed to see how many women (almost one in five) had suffered miscarriages, or had been through the trauma of an abortion (nearly one in six).

And as for me – well, despite my experience of hearing horrendous stories of the darker side of sex, I was taken aback when I realised that the computer print-out showed that very large numbers of the respondents have been *raped* at some time.

Alas, the same is true of *child abuse*. You'll find the statistics on this subject quite horrifying, because quite clearly, childhood sexual abuse has blighted far more women's lives than many people would imagine. And I use the word "blighted" advisedly – because the computer analysis makes it clear that if a woman was a victim of sex abuse as a child, she is appreciably more likely to suffer in adult life from sexual unhappiness and frustration.

Perhaps not surprisingly, there's a similar correlation between rape and subsequent sexual guilt and unhappiness. As you'll see from the figures, the experience of rape is all too likely to foul up a woman's subsequent love-life.

A cheerful picture of late 1980s sex life

Nonetheless, the overall picture of female sexuality revealed by this extraordinary survey is a pretty cheerful one – and that's confirmed by the long personal letters which accompanied so many forms.

I've quoted extensively from those letters, as you'll see in a moment. But please note that the Christian names which I've assigned to respondents' letters are fictitious – though the names of the towns in which the letters were posted are correct.

So, the quite fabulously orgasmic "Suzie of Leeds", quoted below is not actually called "Suzie" though she does come from (and frequently *in*) Leeds.

No, gentlemen I do not have her address. . . .

Now read on. We'll begin by looking at women's "life histories".

Learning about the "facts of life"

We asked the question: "Who (or what) told you about the facts of life?"

In an ideal world, I suppose we'd all learn the facts of life at our mothers' knees (and other low joints).

Seriously, I think that nearly all of us would wish that youngsters learn about sex from some trustworthy and admired person – if not the parents, then a sensible and reliable schoolteacher. Sadly this doesn't appear to be so.

Here is the breakdown of the answers given to the above question:

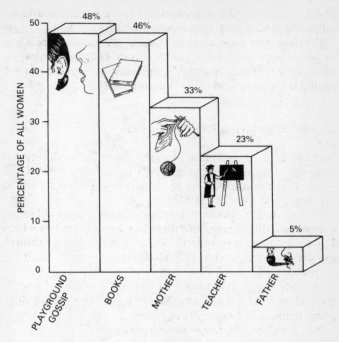

FIG. 2 Where women got the facts of life.

Obviously, many people checked more than one possible answer. But I find it rather depressing that "playground gossip" still comes out as the top source of the facts of life.

And why on earth do only 33% of women report that their mothers told them anything about sex?

Still, there are some grounds for saying that things are improving on the parental front. For when I looked at younger women (those under 20), I found that a much higher percentage of them – 51% in fact – had been told about sex by their mothers.

It's quite clear that whether your mum told you about the birds and the bees or not depends to a considerable extent on what generation you belong to.

You can see what I mean from the next set of figures. They show clearly that the older a woman is, the less likely she is to have had any sex info from her mum. Older women seem to have only very rarely been told anything by their mothers – and seem to have frequently learned "the facts" on their wedding nights.

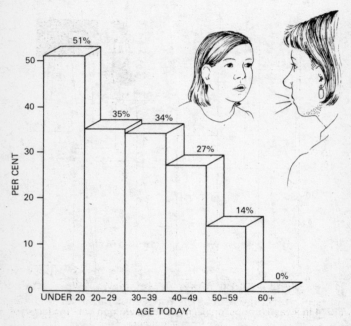

FIG. 3 Most of today's under-20's got "the facts" from their mums – older women rarely did.

So things are getting better where mums are concerned. I wish I could say the same regarding teachers!

I had hoped that school sex education was more widely available these days – and that this would be reflected in a large percentage of younger women saying that they learned something from teacher. Unfortunately, that's not the case. If you look at the figures below, you'll see that the percentage of women who appear to have learned "the facts" in school sex education classes remains amazingly low through the generations.

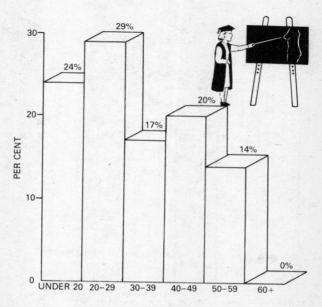

FIG. 4 In all age groups, only a minority of women got "the facts" of life from a teacher.

You may wonder how it varied from generation to generation. After all, there's a widespread belief that "girls are maturing years earlier these days, aren't they?" To hear people talk you'd think that puberty occurs *years* earlier now than it used to.

Well, in fact, the survey shows that the change over the generations has really been very slight. Our results show clearly that the age of onset of periods has not shifted very much over the last forty or fifty years:

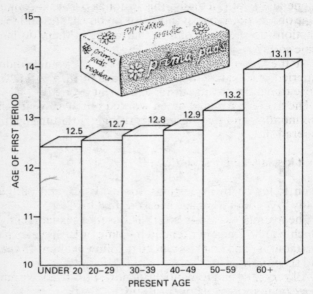

FIG. 5 Age of first period: this hasn't changed a lot over the last 40 to 50 years.

At the present rate of progress, the average age of puberty will not fall below 12 until far into the 21st century. And a good thing too, in my opinion! Young lasses have quite enough to cope with already.

First sexual feelings

I then asked the question: "At what age (approximately) did you first experience sexual feelings?"

As you might expect, most women say that they were in their early teens (12–15) when they first had sexual feelings.

But a slightly surprising 17% say that they experienced such emotions below the age of ten.

An intrepid 2% claim to have had them between the ages of one and five! (Actually, this is not as daft as it sounds, since observations by psychologists on boy babies and their erections do seem to confirm that many of them do have some sort of sexual feelings.)

At the other end of the scale, 2% of women didn't experience sexual feelings until the age of 18. 1% first felt those romantic stirrings at 19, and 1% at over 20.

The average for all women worked out at 13 years and two months, and this varied surprisingly little through the generations.

First kissing, and first petting

Then followed two questions about kissing and petting: firstly "At about what age was your first kiss?"

The average was soon after the onset of sexual feelings, which you'll remember tended to come on at 13 years and two months. The first kiss tended to follow at about 13 years and six months.

All very jolly and romantic. But now, I'm afraid, we must move on to more controversial stuff. . . .

We enquired "At roughly what age did you first go in for sexual petting?"

As long as I can remember, people have had wildly confused views about what constitutes "petting". So in the questionnaire we spelled it out explicitly – as "mutual caressing of the sex organs".

Quite frankly, I'm slightly alarmed to report that among all women the average age of first petting was decidedly younger than many parents would wish – 16 years and four months, in fact.

Not altogether surprisingly, there's a very marked difference in what the various generations reported on this one. As you can see, women over 60 report that they first petted at 22 years and six months. But rather frighteningly, today's teenagers say that on average, they first went in for sexual petting at 14 years and ten months.

Here are the figures:

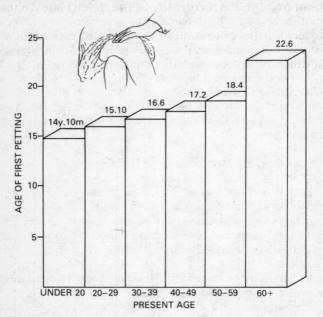

FIG. 6 Age of first "petting" – this is much, much younger today than it used to be.

First intercourse

We asked: "At what age did you first have intercourse?"

I have to be quite blunt and say that I find it quite worrying that the same trend towards earlier and earlier sexual experiment is very clear in this age group, as you can see.

The overall figure for all women was 17¾. But for today's teenagers (the under-20s in Figure Seven), the average came out at a mind-boggling 15 years and 358 days. In short, the average age at which teenage girls are losing their virginity these days appears to be a week before the legal age of consent. I'm sorry, Mrs. Gillick: I don't like it either – but there it is.

Here are the figures which show the "generation effect". As you can see, women over 60 report that on average they didn't lost their virginity till just over the age of 21.

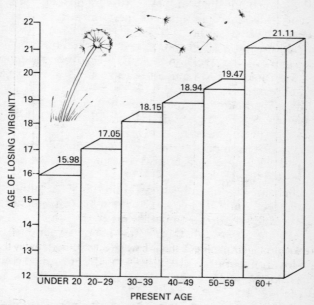

FIG. 7 Age of losing virginity: again, this is much lower in today's young women.

A lot of women wrote letters or notes to say what they felt about that first sexual experience.

Sarah of Thanet said, "I was 18, and I wasn't over-keen. It took him several attempts to complete the breaking of my hymen with his penis. I felt no pain – I just enjoyed the penetration, but not the movement that followed."

Asked if she or the boy had used any contraception, Sarah replied, "No – just ignorance!"

Sarah's experience down in Thanet was actually a bit happier than what many others felt. For instance, Evelyn of Dover said, "I was 17 and single. I was very disappointed. I wasn't sure what was happening."

Eunice of Lancashire just said, "I was 19 and married – and I was sadly disappointed!"

Bronwen of Gwent said, "I was 16. I found it disappointing and I was scared about pregnancy afterwards."

Gayle of Leeds said, "I was 18 and single. I had sex with a married man at a hotel room, having picked him up at a disco that evening. We didn't use any form of contraception because I had had too much to drink, and I was terrified about pregnancy afterwards."

Others had happier experiences the first time: Amanda of Newcastle said, "I was 16. It was OK. And I thought 'Now I know how to do it, I can learn to enjoy it.'"

Emma of Camberwell said, "I was 15 and expected more. I was quite sore afterwards but glad to be rid of virginity. I liked it."

Felicity of Bristol said, "I was 21 and single. I thought it was perfect – and it gave me excitement, rest, liberation and 'linking' – but it's a lot better now!"

Fairly rare was the thoroughly happy experience of Freda of Croydon. She said, "I was 18 and single. It was a very loving experience with a lovely boyfriend – and I count myself lucky. The joy of it will stay with me for the rest of my life."

Like 40% of respondents, (how daft people are!) she didn't use any contraception. Fortunately, she didn't get pregnant.

First orgasm

We next asked: "At roughly what age did you first experience an orgasm?"

Many people (especially men) think that a woman should

start having orgasms as soon as she starts having inter-course. But this is absolute nonsense, of course. This survey shows quite clearly that there's often a gap of some months or even some years between first sex and first orgasm.

Admittedly, this doesn't apply when a woman has reached orgasms through "petting" or through mastur-bation before she has intercourse.

So, as I've said above, the average age of first sex was 17¾. But the average age of first climax was well over two years later – at 19.92 years.

I regard this as one of the most important findings of this survey, because of the fact that so many women worry unnecessarily if they've been making love for a year or two and still haven't reached orgasm. The Delvin Report shows clearly that they are *normal*.

My thanks to Prisca of Stockport, who contributed this graphic (and rather encouraging) account of her first orgasm: "I'd been making love since I was 18, and every time I'd been terribly depressed that I couldn't come. I took lover after lover. By the time I'd reached 28, I'd slept with at least thirty men – result: absolute zilch. But one Christ-mas when I was going on 29, I was in bed with the man I eventually married. It was so warm and close and tender that I felt wonderfully relaxed. And all of a sudden, when he was kissing my clitoris I felt something like a warm flame rising inside me until it burst like a bombshell and I hugged his head and said, 'I love you!' Since then, I've never looked back."

Good for you, Prisca of Stockport. It took you ten years, but by golly you made it.

Masturbation

Now let's turn to the ticklish subject of masturbation. As I said in the introduction, this is a topic that people – particularly women – don't like to talk about. Indeed, when I first mentioned female masturbation in print some years

31

ago, I got some really aggressive letters saying that (for instance): "ladies don't do such things"; "if they do, they're no ladies"; furthermore, "the chaps at our club (*seriously*) reckon that it would be bad for a girl's health . . .".

Well, my word: does this survey dispel all the old myths about DIY? It surely does.

In fact, I think that here the survey makes a very important contribution to the study of the sexuality of the British female. For it reveals that the vast majority (92.4%) of all the respondents have masturbated at some time or other.

The average age of starting was 15.67 years. Furthermore a staggering 85% of respondents do it *now*. Even I find that slightly surprising, when you consider that the majority of the women who filled in the Delvin Report questionnaire are either married, or living together, or have a steady boy friend.

But 83% of married women reported "I'm still doing it!"

Furthermore, three-quarters of all women appear to do it to bring themselves to orgasm – the figures being the same for married women.

However, these ladies are not necessarily having to go in for a spot of solitary DIY to make up for their spouses' inadequacies. In fact, the answers of many women make clear that they actually masturbate not by themselves but *during love-making* with their partners.

43% of all women say that they've done this as part of love-play with their husbands. For instance, Margot of Edinburgh wrote: "To get my husband going, I strip off in front of him and then sensuously rub myself until I've reached my first climax. Then, and only then, I let him touch me, by which time he's absolutely desperate to get his hands on me!"

Attitudes to female masturbation among women themselves are clearly pretty liberal. Only 5% of all women think it is "wrong" these days – and that free-and-easy attitude is pretty much the same across the generations – though 8% of the 40–49 age group think it's wrong.

Interestingly, virtually 100% of over-60s thought it was

morally OK – which perhaps reflects the fact that so many women in this age group find it a solace and comfort.

How women rate their sex lives today

How do you rate your own sex lives? I'm delighted to say that most of you are pretty happy with the way things are going for you in bed.

71% of the women who replied rated their love lives as being "good", "very good", or even "excellent". But this means that 29% replied "poor", "awful" or "non-existent".

The women who *didn't* rate their sex lives as up to much did quite often have significant "danger factors" in their past lives – for instance, a past history of rape or childhood sexual abuse. More about this worrying finding towards the end of this chapter.

The two groups who were most likely to rate their sex lives as excellent were the under-20s and the over-50s. I must say, I find that latter statistic very encouraging indeed!

In our study of major British cities, women from Leeds were the most likely to rate their sex lives as "excellent". Once again, I have no idea why this should be so.

How many times per week?

Ah, this is the question that all sex surveys ask, isn't it? And it's the one that always fascinates people – because they want to see how their own bedtime performances compare with those of other folk.

But before I give the results, just a word of warning. If the number of times that YOU make love per week is less than the average, for Heaven's sake don't start thinking you're abnormal or inadequate or something.

Just as human beings vary in height, so too they vary in the frequency with which they have intercourse. Furthermore, the number of times per week that you "do it" is not really what matters. It's quality (not quantity) that counts.

33

Anyway, now to the figures. The average number of times per week was a remarkable 3.91. "Remarkable", because this is appreciably above the 2.4 times a week which has been quoted as the norm for many years.

So either Britain is getting sexier – or else those who responded to the survey are an unusually randy lot! (Personally, I suspect that both statements may well be true. . . .)

By the way, in our light-hearted mini-survey of large towns and cities, Leeds women again came out top, "doing it" 4.8 times a week on average – in the course of which they clocked up 5.95 orgasms. Preeminent among them was the amazing Suzie – of whom more in a moment.

How many orgasms per week?

That brings us to the subject of "How many orgasms do you have a week?"

Once again, can I interject a word of warning? If you are enjoying your own personal sex life, then it doesn't matter two hoots if you only have one orgasm every six months. So when you read about the orgasmic exploits of Suzie of Leeds (see below) please don't feel that you are somehow inferior to her. For all I know, you may be a very great deal happier than Suzie. . . .

So, to the orgasmic results!

Women report that they have 5.47 orgasms per week (though I don't suppose that the odd 0.47 is really a lot of fun). Many respondents have *multiple* orgasms during a love-making/love play session – which is something I'll discuss further in a moment.

In addition, many climaxes are actually achieved through "petting" – or through self-stimulation (as we've seen in the section on masturbation). The additional notes and letters which people have sent in make this very clear. Anne of Cardiff says: "I have put myself down for seven orgasms a week. In fact, I only get to see my fiancé once a week, and would expect to have one climax with him through petting,

34

and one during intercourse. But I'm afraid I do have a very passionate nature and get frustrated the rest of the week. So I do bring myself to a climax before I fall asleep every night except on Sundays, because I have an early start on Monday mornings."

What amazingly well-planned sex lives they seem to lead in Cardiff. *Cymru am byth*!

Not surprisingly, the highest orgasmic rates are found among women who rate their love lives as "excellent". They record an average of 7½ climaxes a week.

But it's interesting that among this highly-satisfied group of women who say that their sex lives are excellent, a substantial minority appear to be having either just one orgasm a week, or none at all.

So I think this does prove what I said above: *that it's perfectly possible to enjoy an excellent sex life without setting world records for orgasms.*

And talking about world records for orgasms, next on the agenda comes (and I use the word advisedly) the amazing Suzie of Leeds.

Now I cannot be absolutely sure whether Suzie's pulling my leg or not, but I don't think she is. (Just in case, I didn't include her claims in the main survey.) But if she's telling the truth, her orgasmic score is really quite phenomenal.

She claims to be a Yorkshire schoolteacher in her late 30s. According to the letter clipped to her form, she has several lovers and a husband ("He's away a lot . . .").

Suzie says: "Although my professional colleagues think of me as 'the quiet type', I just seem to have a terrific appetite for sex, especially about two weeks after a period. I try if possible to have sex with my husband, or with a lover, or by myself, every night, except when I've got the curse. As I can achieve around twenty orgasms in every session, that gives me about 140 climaxes a week! *Awful*, isn't it?"

Well Suzie, I prefer to regard you as a sort of female Geoff Boycott – knocking up a weekly century for Yorkshire.

And I must admit that Suzie's alleged total of 140 climaxes a week is a physiological possibility (see Chapter Nine) though admittedly a rather enervating one. For as we'll see in the section on multiple climaxes, there certainly is quite a substantial minority of women who can rattle off twenty orgasms in an evening. However, to do this seven nights in a row would (I feel) leave one with scant energy for schoolteaching. . . .

More "orgasmic" questions

And now on to the further questions which we asked about that perennial subject of interest – orgasms.

As you'll have read above, we've already established that on average, respondents started having orgasms at age 19.92 years, and that they have about 5.47 a week! (And do you realise that for a 50-year-old lady, that means that she's probably clocked up about 8,533 climaxes in the last thirty years or so. . . .)

But we also asked quite a few more questions about women's orgasmic responses.

First, we asked the simple query: "Have you ever experienced a sexual climax?"

94% of respondents said "yes"; 6% said "no".

The next thing to establish was "Do you reach a climax nowadays?" (We made it clear that we meant either during petting or intercourse.)

Here the scores aren't quite so high. The replies went as in Figure 8 opposite.

So you can see that the myth – perpetuated by raunchy novels – that women *always* reach a climax is just a load of old rhubarb! Just 17% of our respondents (about one in six) always have an "org" during petting or intercourse. And only 65% reach it "always or most times".

This brings us to the important question of *climax during intercourse*. I've been saying for years that (contrary to popular belief) most women don't always reach an orgasm during actual intercourse – and that if you can regularly ring

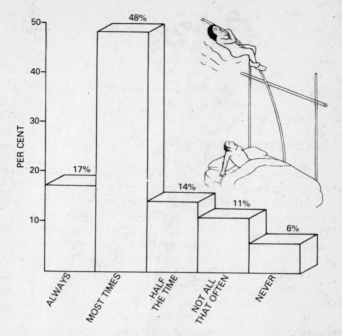

FIG. 8 Do you reach a climax nowadays (during either petting or intercourse)? Only 6% of women said "Never".

the bell *with your man actually inside you*, then you're doing very well indeed.

Our results make this point clear to anyone who doubted it. As you can see from the figures below, the proportion of women who *always* reach a climax during actual intercourse is small – scarcely more than one in eight, in fact.

Even those who reach it "always or most times" during actual intercourse are in a slight minority of 49.7%.

I note with interest that married women, and also women who described their sex lives as "extremely good", were more likely to have climaxes with their partners inside them.

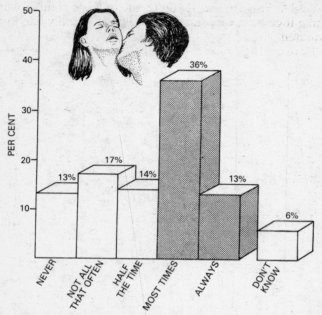

FIG. 9 Do you reach a climax during intercourse itself? Slightly less than half of all women say they usually do.

This brings us to the question of "simultaneous climax" – so beloved of fiction writers, and (in my view) unrealistically so!

For the survey bears out my oft-expressed contention that simultaneous orgasms are not really very common, and that couples who achieve them can count themselves jolly lucky!

As you can see from Figure 10, more than one in four of all respondents say that a simultaneous orgasm simply *never* happens, and a further 46% say that it only happens "occasionally".

A mere 14% of respondents say that they "almost always" achieve simultaneous climax with their partners.

And as you can see, if you're one of those couples who come together every time – well, you're literally one in a hundred!

Here are the figures:

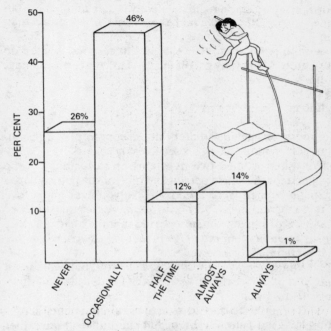

FIG. 10 Do you come together? Only 1 in 100 couples "always" do this.

To close our orgasmic section, let's turn to that question of *multiple* orgasms. 60% of respondents said that they could reach multiple climaxes; 33% said they couldn't; and 7% said they didn't know.

Actually, that last answer is not as daft as it sounds – because some women experience a sort of long drawn out or "serial" orgasm with lots of little peaks. Naturally, this is difficult to distinguish from true multiple orgasms.

Encouragingly, more "mature" women are decidedly more likely to be able to have multiple orgasms. And some intrepid over-40s have indicated that they can sometimes clock up fifteen or even twenty orgasms at a session. Furthermore, among the relatively small number of 60-plus, a sparkling 89% said they could do it more than once.

So it appears to be true that in this respect, women do have more fun as they get older. . . . Isn't that encouraging, ladies?

Adultery

To be serious again: adultery does seem to play a prominent part in many women's sex lives these days.

We asked women two questions on this subject – one designed for the single person and one for the married one.

Single women were asked: "Have you ever made love with a married man?" It is with some regret that I record that 39% of single women reported that they had. *In other words, virtually four out of ten of the single women said that they'd committed adultery*.

This finding may seem surprising to you, but is in fact in line with other recent surveys on the incidence of adultery in British women.

It's not my business to make moral comments in this book but I must say that I'd be happier if there were rather fewer young single women having it orf (as we say at the General Medical Council) with married blokes.

Now, *married* women were asked the following question about adultery: "Have you ever been unfaithful?"

37% of those who are currently married said they'd committed adultery at some time – again *not far off four out of every ten*.

This figure may sound bad (particularly if you're a husband), but it's actually a bit less than the figures reported by a couple of other recent British surveys. What my survey and the other recent ones do seem to show is that adultery by married women is much commoner than it was a generation ago.

Not surprisingly, the percentage of women who report having been unfaithful is appreciably higher in the "divorced, separated and widowed" group. 53% of these said that they'd been unfaithful to a husband in the past.

Women's relationship with men

Let's have a look at the questions which dealt with relationships with men – and with *their* attitudes to women nowadays.

This was the first questions we asked: "Are you happy with your (male) partner's (or partners') attitude to love-making?"

68% said yes – which is good. But a whopping 23% said no – which is bad.

Surprisingly, younger women and women who are living with a bloke are the most likely to be happy with their guys' attitude to sex. Those who were most likely to be unhappy with their male partners included women over 40 – and of course, women who rated their sex lives as "poor".

Complaints about male partners' attitudes varied wildly. Many women said something like "He just doesn't bother to be romantic" (this came very often from middle-aged women) or "He can't be bothered to take the trouble to make sure that I reach a climax too." This was so common as to be epidemic.

Sarah of Thanet voiced quite a common complaint when she wrote: "If I don't make the first move, then he doesn't either, so nothing gets done. (And neither do I.)"

The next (and related) question was this: "Men are sometimes said to be more gentle and understanding these days. Do you think that, where sex is concerned, the men you've come into contact with have changed very much in recent years?"

Well, I'm afraid that only 38% of women thought that men had changed. 40% thought that they *hadn't* – while a surprisingly high 22% (perhaps stupefied by the question) said "Don't know".

Single women were rather more likely than married ones to believe that men have changed.

Not surprisingly, the strongest opposition to any idea that men have altered for the better came from the "divorced, separated and widowed" group – and also from women who recorded their own sex lives as "awful" or "non-existent".

A member of both these categories is Jeannie of Belfast, who wrote – with amazing alliterative power, "Blokes are a bunch of bastards, and always will be."

Clearly, the "New Man" has so far only established a modest beach-head in the UK. . . .

On a slightly lighter note, we asked a couple of questions about how women viewed men's physical as opposed to emotional characteristics.

First of all, we asked: "Is the size of your partner's sex organ important to you?"

Now like most doctors who write about sex, I get vast numbers of letters from chaps who feel that their penises are on the small side. Our traditional reply is: "Don't worry, old boy – women aren't interested in the size of your John Thomas."

Well, just recently several women have taken me to task for this rather smug attitude – which was one reason why I included the question in the survey.

And the remarkable results do appear to show that agony uncles and aunties have tended to be a bit too complacent about this one! For virtually one woman in three (32%) said "*Yes* – the size of a partner's sex organ is important to me."

"I like a chap to have a bit of bulk," said the engagingly frank Christine of Pinner. However just over two-thirds (67%) did say that the size of a guy's organ isn't important.

And gentlemen who are worried that they're a bit on the under-endowed side will be relieved to hear the response we got to our next question: "Do you feel happy about the size of your own partner's sex organ?"

Happily, a whopping 94% said "yes" to this one. Interestingly, the only group who weren't so keen on saying "yes" were those women who rate their own sex lives as "awful" or "non-existent".

At the end of our survey, we also asked readers a final cheeky question about their menfolk's physical characteristics:

Which parts of a man's body do you find
(a) most attractive?
(b) least attractive?

"Men's feet" were "least favourite" most often. And the most popular part of a man? Not what you gents might think. "Men's bottoms" appear to lead the field! P'raps this enthusiasm for male buttocks isn't surprising. For as Mary from Kent says: "A chap's bum is what we like to cling onto while we're making love!"

Rape and child abuse

Now we come on to a much more disturbing aspect of women's relationships with males – the twin topics of rape and childhood sexual abuse (which, let's make no bones about it, is almost always committed by men).

The figures for rape in the Delvin Report are absolutely devastating. When they first came back from the computer, I couldn't believe them. Yet in fact, high as they are, they are very much in line with what Rape Crisis and feminist organisations have been claiming recently.

Virtually one in ten of all respondents (9.9%) reported that they have been raped. The figures were particularly bad in the under-20s – 13% of whom say that they have been rape victims.

And there's worse. Rape seems to have had an appalling effect on the subsequent sexual happiness of these poor women. Almost half of all rape victims report that their sex lives are now "poor", "awful" or "non-existent". And an abnormally high proportion of them have ended up with wrecked marriages.

I accept that you can't carelessly extrapolate from these figures and say with certainty that "almost 10% of the female population of Britain have been raped". For one thing, an obvious defect of my survey is that a woman who has been the victim of rape may be more likely than the average female to send in a completed form to the Delvin Report, to express her outrage.

On the other hand, you could argue that a rape victim might be *less* likely to take part in a sex survey of this sort – which was basically intended to be light-hearted and good fun.

Whatever the truth, I think that the mere fact that so many women have written in saying that they have been raped (and that their subsequent sex lives have been pretty disastrous) is profoundly disturbing.

The figures for *childhood sex abuse* are also appalling.

I found it hard to believe the initial computer record – but the print-out is quite definite.

Very nearly one in five (18%) of all women who took part in this survey say that they were sexually abused as children.

The sad little messages attached to these questionnaires speak of being interfered with by grandfathers, uncles, family friends (male) – and even fathers.

And (just as with rape), the outcome of all this is clear. Women who have been molested as children are far more likely to report that their present-day sex lives are terrible. Indeed, 26% of those who now have an "awful" or "non-existent" sex life were sexually molested as little girls. Similarly, there appears to be evidence that women who were interfered with as children are more likely to suffer marriage break-up.

The only slightly brighter spot in this truly depressing section of the report is a faint indication that child sex abuse may actually be getting a little less common (which is not what you'd think judging by recent newspaper reports).

While a staggering 27% of women in the 40 to 60 age group reported that they had suffered from it, only (*only!*)

16% of today's teenagers have run into that particular kind of trouble.

So it may be that the incidence of child sex abuse has lessened just a little over the last thirty or forty years. More studies are clearly needed in order to find out.

Changing sexual behaviour

My feeling is that after years of permissiveness, we're just seeing the start of a swing back of the pendulum – mainly caused by fear of AIDS, herpes, cancer of the cervix and so on.

So we asked the readers to say whether these alarming reports of sex diseases had recently made them alter their own sexual behaviour.

More than one in four (27%, actually) said "yes". The highest rates were among the single women, among "co-habiting" women, and among women who rated their sex lives as "awful" or "non-existent".

Not surprisingly, married women weren't so likely to feel the urge to change their sexual practices – only 20% said they would. *And worryingly, remarkably few teenagers (only 18%) have so far opted to modify their sexual habits.* This is frightening.

My belief is that these figures are likely to increase dramatically in the next year or two, as people realise the full horror of the AIDS outbreak.

Sex between women

Finally, let's move to the section of the Delvin Report which dealt with the question of sex between women.

The first question we asked on this subject was: "Do you regard yourself as straight, gay or bisexual?"

As this survey was so clearly directed at investigation of sexual relationships with men, I didn't really expect that many lesbians would take the trouble to plough through it.

And that expectation appears to have been right. Virtually no one ticked the "gay" box – even though it is generally reckoned that at least 5% of the female population are basically lesbian.

But it was a very different matter with bisexuality! I've been saying for a long time that there are far more bisexual people around than is generally recognised. And our survey seems to bear this out. *No less than one in twelve of all the women who responded described themselves as bisexual.*

Bisexuality was commonest in the 20–29 age group, and least common in those women who are married. (But even among married women, it's one in twenty.)

Rather more startling were the results of our questions about past sexual experiences with other women. *Virtually a fifth of all respondents said that they had had a sexual affair with another female.*

This may seem amazing to you. But in fact, a little-known finding of the Kinsey Report (back in 1953) was that as many as 30% of all US college girls had had such a relationship. So perhaps things haven't changed all that much in thirty-three years.

How orgasmic were these relationships? Well, of the respondents who said that they'd had a lesbian affair, 43% said that it had progressed to the stage of orgasm.

The obvious conclusion from this section of the questionnaire is that many women do have a brief physical relationship with another female at some time in their lives. But this seems in most cases to be a passing phase, and they frequently settle down to a heterosexual way of life.

Certainly, I can find nothing definite in the figures to suggest that these women are damaged by the experience, though it's noticeable that they seem to be slightly more likely than average to choose to live with a man, rather than get married.

Also, there does seem to be slight tendency for women who've had lesbian experiences to report that their present-day sex lives are poor. But the trend is not strong. Much more typical is the story of Amanda of Greater Manchester who notes: "I had a very sexy affair with my room-mate while I was at university, mostly stroking and oral sex. But after three months, we both realised that we were basically into guys – and that was the end of it. I don't know about her, but I'm now happily married with a baby, and I wouldn't really fancy another woman any more."

CHAPTER THREE

Aiming For One-Partner Sex – And "Relieving The Monogamy"

How many sex partners have most people had? ● Why is it difficult to get people to keep to one partner? ● What happens if you don't ● Diane's frightening case history ● The terrifying "AIDS Chain" ● "Serial" partners are better than promiscuity ● "Relieving the monogamy": some ways of making one-partner sex a lot of fun

How many sex partners have most people had?

There are a few men (and, indeed a few women) who have had sex with literally hundreds of different partners.

But most people aren't as daft as that (and "daft" really is the word for it – if you have sex with hundreds of different people, you're almost bound to pick up something serious – and there's an increasing likelihood that that "something serious" will be AIDS).

In fact, the Delvin Report suggests that the average late 1980s woman has only had about *four to six* male partners in her life.

Slightly worryingly, the figures are decidedly higher for *young* women: these days, 22% of girls have already clocked up about four partners before they leave their teens. A girl who goes on at this rate will obviously have been bedded by several dozen blokes by the time she's 30.

Are men any worse? Figures for *men* which have been

recently obtained by my excellent fellow (if that's the right word) "agony auntie" Deidre Sanders suggest that at the present time, the average British male is only slightly more promiscuous. She says that:

★A quarter of young adult males have only had one lover;
★A third have had up to five lovers;
★A fifth have had up to eleven lovers;
★Another fifth of all young gents claim to have had eleven or more girls.

Now these figures are perhaps not *sensationally* high. But they do give a clear indication that nowadays the average person simply doesn't go in for the "one sex partner for life" principle which has been held up as a shining example throughout the Christian era.

And though the *average* number of partners for both sexes is fairly low, the fact is that a sizeable proportion of men and women do "score" higher than the average, and make love with almost anyone attractive whom they can persuade into bed.

For instance, as this book was being completed, it was being reported in British newspapers that some young English girls on holiday in Spain were cheerfully "bonking" (to use the current vogue word) with as many as fourteen different blokes in a fortnight's holiday – one a night, in fact!

Similarly, my *She* magazine survey shows quite clearly that 2% of female readers say that they have had more than 100 lovers in a lifetime. (Good Heavens!)

All of which indicates that people find it very, very difficult to pick just one sexual partner – and to stick to him (or her) throughout life.

Why is it difficult to get people to keep to one partner?

There are several reasons why it's so hard to get human beings to opt for "one-partner sex".

49

Firstly, you have to bear in mind the fact that "one-partner sex" is completely contrary to the lessons which the human race has learned in a million years of evolution.

Let me explain. A million years ago, there were just a handful of human beings on the Earth, battling to stay alive in a very hostile environment.

For a very long period of time, your tribe was likely to die out if you didn't reproduce pretty quickly. So, the simple evolutionary fact is that *it was people who were very keen on sex who were most likely to have descendants*. Therefore, we are all descended from some extremely randy ancestors – who have passed down a good deal of this general raunchiness to today's human beings!

And I'm afraid that the more *promiscuous* a prehistoric male was, the more likely he'd be to pass on his wicked ways to subsequent generations. Men who went round impregnating vast numbers of prehistoric women were of course very likely to have surviving children. Men who kept to one partner *weren't*!

The strong tendency of males to be promiscuous has continued to the present day – despite all the efforts of religion and the Law (but only during the last 2,000 years or so) to make men monogamous. It's an unfortunate fact of life that deep down, many males (probably most) would really prefer to have as many women as possible!

It seems to be generally agreed by sociologists that women are *not* so promiscuous by nature – though there are some authorities on sex who say that "given an equal opportunity, women are as enthusiastic as men about embracing a large number of partners".

Certainly, there's no doubt that in the last thirty years women do seem to have become much more likely to go in for promiscuity and infidelity.

One factor in causing this must surely have been the availability of (almost) totally safe contraception from the 1960s onwards.

Admittedly, the "Permissive Society" seems to have

started very shortly *before* the Pill and the IUD became generally available.

But anyone who lived through the "Swinging Sixties" will remember that vast numbers of women seemed to suddenly realise that the fact that they were safe from unwanted pregnancy meant that they could go to party after party with every intention of finding a man – and taking him home to bed.

Habits like that are not all that easy to break – so perhaps it's not surprising that today's surveys suggest that about four out of ten wives have been unfaithful to their husbands.

Indeed, it appears that today's women are finding it almost as difficult as men are to keep to a solitary partner for the rest of their lives.

What happens if you don't keep to one partner?

Well, you may get away with it, of course!

But it has to be accepted that "multi-partner sex" does carry certain very appreciable risks. These are:

★Unwanted pregnancy – often by the wrong partner;
★Emotional problems;
★Marriage break-up;
★Minor sex infections;
★VD;
★And – alas! – AIDS.

As we approach the "Nervous Nineties", I'm afraid that more and more people are going to find that an agreeable night of romance away from their regular partner is going to have the kind of appalling results described below.

Diane's frightening case history

Diane was one of the first heterosexuals to acquire the AIDS virus in Britain.

By today's standards, she was a pretty "straightlaced" sort of girl: two previous lovers when she was about 19, and a long term relationship with Bill – the man she intended to marry.

Diane decided to have a brief ski-ing holiday before getting formally engaged. At an *après-ski* party she met a nice young chap and (under the genial influence of *glühwein* and Austrian music) thought "Well – why not have one last fling?"

She spent the night with him, and never saw him again. A few months later, she was HIV positive – and a few months after that, she was dead.

Her fiancé is now HIV positive too (having acquired the infection from her) and he, poor man, is waiting to see if his fate will be the same.

The terrifying AIDS chain

If that young man sleeps with anybody else (which I hope he won't) then he'd probably – though not certainly – pass the virus to them, and the terrifying AIDS chain would continue.

It's worth looking at this "AIDS chain" in some detail. The simple drawing opposite shows just how the "chain" works – and how vast numbers of people can be infected in a very short time.

In Stage One, (at the top of the drawing) John, who is one of the hundreds of thousands of bisexual men in Britain, catches the virus without realising it.

In Stage Two, he gives it to Jenny during a one-night stand.

In Stage Three, Jenny (who has no idea anything is wrong with her) gives it to her husband Jeremy.

Unfortunately, Jeremy is more than fond of what gents tend to call "a bit on the side". In Stage Four, over a period of a year, he has sex with half a dozen other girls – five of whom catch the virus from him.

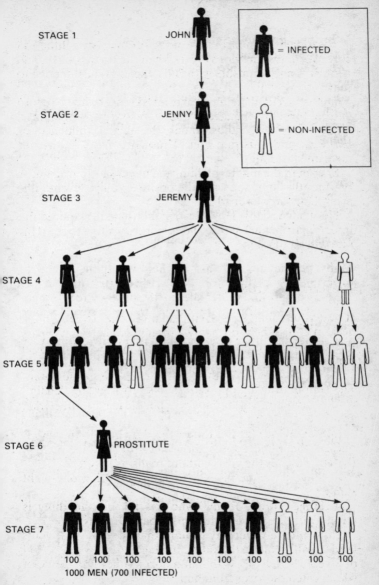

FIG. 11 The AIDS chain

In Stage Five, those girls each sleep with two or three boy friends. Most of those men get it.

In Stage Six, the infected men may pass the virus to their various girl friends and wives. Worse still, one of those men goes with a prostitute – and infects her.

Over the next year, she sleeps with 1,000 clients (quite a small number for a prostitute) – and infects over 700 of them. . . .

And so it will go on, and on, and on. Condoms will prevent some of this spread – but not all of it. Unless our society can manage to give up the easy-going (and admittedly often very pleasant) promiscuity of the last thirty years, we are in terrible, terrible trouble!

"Serial" partners are better than promiscuity

Many people do feel that in their youth they need to experiment sexually before they settle down in life.

Many others find rather later in life that they're no longer happy with their original partner, and seek sexual solace elsewhere.

This needn't mean disaster for them. For if you take care to stick to *just one partner at a time*, you will at least cut down greatly on your risk of catching AIDS.

You can never be *entirely* safe, of course. But a man or woman who practises "serial monogamy" (that is trying at least to be faithful to the current partner) is much less likely to acquire this awful virus.

Obviously, it also helps if you can pick a partner who's *also* practising "serial monogamy"! For if you choose someone who's a bit promiscuous, then clearly your own risks of getting AIDS must go up immediately.

For what we have to remember in these worrying times is this. WHEN YOU HAVE SEX WITH SOMEBODY THESE DAYS, IN EFFECT YOU'RE HAVING SEX WITH ALL THEIR RECENT PARTNERS AS WELL.

So the only *completely* safe sex is really monogamous sex.

"Relieving the monogamy": some ways of making one-partner sex a lot of fun

So, you're going to try and be monogamous?

Don't panic! It needn't be as dull as it sounds. Couples all over the world who've opted for this "new morality" are finding that – with a little application – "home matches" can be more fun, more fulfilling, more loving, more reliable, and of course *safer* than "away fixtures".

And how do they achieve this?

Well, the key word is ROMANCE.

Romance is the most important factor in any monogamous partnership – the thing that keeps it from being boring, tedious and repetitious. I can't emphasise strongly enough that *any partnership will almost certainly fail if the romance goes out of it.*

So here are a few helpful tips, based on the word "romance". Use them to keep the sparkle in *your* partnership:

"R" is to remind you that there are times when you need to be rollicking; randy; raunchy; or possibly even ravished! But most of all, "R" stands for *relationship*: that's what you have to work at if you want to keep it all together. OK, you may both be terrific in bed; you may have the most devastating flickering tongue, the most reliable erection, or the most indefatigable right hand in the business; but you will *not* achieve happy monogamy if your basic relationship is wrong. Sort it out – or you're in trouble.

"O" is to remind you about orgasms (don't forget to give your partner some); oral sex (ditto); and 'ormones (sorry about that). But most of all, "O" is for *"originality"*; don't be repetitive, boring and predictable in your relationship with him or her. Keep thinking of new and interesting things to do – and do them! And they needn't be *sexual* things either – what about surprising him/her with a gift of a single rose, delivered out of the blue by special messenger? (Yes, it can be done quite cheaply: contact Unirose Gift

55

Service, 125 Askew Road, London W12 9AV – telephone 01-749 9735.)

"**M**" is for multiple climaxes (you may not want them yourself – but at least consider the *possibility* that your partner might want to do it more than once!); mutual caressing; masturbation (something which can actually help quite a lot of relationships – see Chapter Two); but most of all, for *mind*.

You ignore your partner's mind at your peril. If you treat him or her as just a sex object – something to give you an orgasm when you feel like it – your relationship is doomed to failure. Try exploring his/her mind: to be quite honest, you'll find it more use than any sex manual.

"**A**" is for adultery (*not* a great idea: four out of ten people do it, but it's best avoided if you can); aphrodisiacs (a waste of time); and adventure (*not* a waste of time – when did you last try using a) ice cubes, b) baby oil, c) champagne in your love-making?).

Most of all though, "A" stands for *"affirmation"* – which means boosting your partner's confidence by supporting and praising him or her, paying him/her little compliments, and trying to back him/her up through the crises of life. A little affirmation can do an awful lot in helping a couple stay together long-term.

"**N**" is for nipples (remember – they're an erogenous zone in *both* sexes!); nostalgia (a potent force in keeping a relationship going – when did the two of you last visit the place where you first met?); nickers (well, very nearly); and most of all, *naughtiness*. What too many couples forget is the need for a spot of naughtiness in their relationship: naughty underwear, naughty week-ends, naughty sex games – all the slightly "wicked" things that put a certain *risqué* sparkle into a sexual relationship!

"**C**" is for clitoris (which nearly all men need to pay more attention to); climaxes (see Chapter Nine); cherishing (very important); but most of all, *cuddling*. Studies show that what many women – and a heck of a lot of men – want most is to be cuddled. It's no good coming home and using the most advanced techniques to extract an orgasm from your partner if you don't cuddle him or her beforehand and afterwards – and preferably "during" as well.

And finally **"E"** is for education (learn more about love-making, and it'll pay you both rich dividends); enthusiasm; erection (just to stress that you don't need it every time – a couple can have great fun without it); eroticism (never hesitate to use anything erotic that you both like); and ecstasy.

Oh yes, and above all there's *enjoyment*. It's meant to be fun: not an Olympic event! If you concentrate on enjoying sex together (rather than striving for "performance"), you won't go far wrong.

Note: if you need more help, you may be interested to know that one result of the AIDS threat is that there are actually now *courses* for couples who want to learn to stay faithful and avoid seeking sex elsewhere. Write (enclosing s.a.e.) to: The Institute of Marital Studies, The Tavistock Centre, Belsize Lane, London, NW3 5BA.

CHAPTER FOUR

Multi-Partner Sex – And Its Risks

What the Delvin Report revealed about multi-partner sex • Brenda's disastrous story • Adultery • Sex parties and orgies (and the rival Harley Street mobs) • Threesomes (troilism) • Open marriages • Wife swapping • Prostitution

What the Delvin Report revealed about multi-partner sex

Let me just make clear what I mean by "multi-partner sex". This means *having more than one sexual relationship going at a time*.

As we've seen in the last chapter, that's far more dangerous than having a string of lovers (or husbands or wives) *one after the other*. If you have two or more relationships going at the same time, I'm afraid that you greatly increase your chances of getting (and spreading) AIDS or other less serious conditions.

So, "multi-partner sex" includes such things as:

★Having two or more lovers at once;
★Being unfaithful to your spouse;
★Going in for "threesomes";
★Wife-swapping;
★Going to sex parties, orgies and "key-parties", and so on.

Now, how common is multi-partner sex? Well, unfortunately (human beings being what they are), it's very common indeed.

Exact figures are hard to obtain. But in the Delvin Report survey we found, for instance, that almost four out of ten wives said that they had had an adulterous relationship with another man while still (presumably) making love with their husbands.

Other recent surveys suggest that a similar proportion of British husbands have attempted the (often physically demanding!) task of having affairs with other women while still making love to their wives.

What about *single* people? Well, I'm afraid that the years I spent in the consulting room rapidly opened my eyes to the fact that it's become more or less the norm for young, single men and women to "run" several partners at once. When problems like (say) thrush arose, we frequently found ourselves treating a girl's three regular boy friends – and sometimes *their* other girl friends as well.

In the Delvin Report survey, we found that 25% of women reported that they had had seven or more lovers – often keeping two or three "on the go" at once. A typical example was Paula of Birmingham who wrote this brief "sex history":

"*Age 20* – lost virginity with Stephen. Not much fun.
Age 21 – tried it again with John. Much better!
Age 22 to 24 – slept regularly with John, Mark and Mick. Also occasionally with Stephen. He *still* wasn't much fun.
Age 25 – still sleeping with John and Mick. (Mark faded out of picture.) Met Stavros – fabulous! Stavros found out I was sleeping with John and Mick – trouble! John and Mick faded out of picture too – rapidly, as Stavros is rather large."

Quite so. In fact, Paula's story of multi-partner sex is really very tame by today's standards. There are in fact quite a few women who've succumbed to the temptation to make love with several blokes *in a single evening* – which really is "chancing your arm" (if you got pregnant, you'd obviously have no idea who the father was).

You may imagine that this kind of thing is very rare. But in fact, the Delvin Report found that *almost one in six women said they'd had intercourse with more than one man in the course of an evening*.

Admittedly, 60% of women said they would never do such a thing. But a surprising 23% said "I might".

We'll find out more in a moment about British women's attitudes to such exotic activities as threesomes, orgies and wife-swapping. But first let's look at a fairly typical case history of a girl who dabbled unwisely in multi-boy friend sex – and, I'm afraid, came badly unstuck.

Brenda's disastrous story

Brenda was a nurse at a teaching hospital. She was also a "child of the Sixties" – in other words, she'd come into adulthood at a time when a spot of "free love" and pot-smoking (often both at the same time) were suddenly there for the taking.

Brenda more or less decided that she was going to "run" two or three boy friends at once until she was ready for marriage. She felt that as long as she didn't have *more* than about three chaps on the go at once, she "wasn't being promiscuous".

And she stuck to her own "rules" for several years – only once transgressing, on a memorable but decidedly unwise night when she went to a party, got both tipsy *and* "stoned", and finished up by obliging no less than eight chaps in the bathroom.

Brenda understandably put that episode out of her mind when she eventually got married. But one of her former lovers (perhaps one of the gents in the bathroom – who knows?) had left her with more than an erotic memory. *She found that she was totally unable to have children.*

Like literally tens of thousands of young women who

went through the 60s, 70s or 80s, she'd been unlucky enough to end up with her tubes totally blocked by an unnoticed infection.

We know now what we didn't know back in the 1960s – that this very common form of infertility is caused by a very widespread germ called "chlamydia". (It's described in Chapter Eight.)

Vast numbers of people carry it in their sexual "plumbing" – mostly without realising it. And unfortunately for Brenda, she'd slept with one of them.

P.S. In case you're interested, Brenda's infertility wasn't really treatable. But things didn't turn out too badly, as she and her husband adopted two very sweet children.

Adultery

Adultery, as we've seen above, is awfully common in Britain today. In many social groups, it's so accepted as to scarcely raise people's eyebrows.

The Delvin Report found that four out of ten *single* women had committed adultery with a married man.

And as I've said above, a similar proportion of *married* women have been unfaithful to their husbands.

Indeed the percentage of wives who've committed adultery is now very nearly as high as the proportion of husbands who've done it. (This is a very big change from the 1950s, when adultery by wives seems to have been much rarer.)

Why do people commit adultery? Studies indicate that they give two main reasons, one of which is surprisingly mundane. Here they are:

1. *The opportunity just presented itself*

Among men, this reason is the commonest, according to Deidre Sanders' recent survey of British males. It's a sad fact that remarkably few blokes seem to be able to resist temptation when they're offered the chance of going to bed with a pretty woman – particularly if there's a reasonable prospect (e.g. on a business trip away from home) that they won't be found out.

Many women also commit adultery practically on impulse – because "the opportunity just presented itself". Very often, they succumb because the occasion seems wonderfully romantic, rather than particularly sexy.

And of course, in both sexes these "opportunist" acts of adultery often happen because the person's resistance has been lowered by alcohol (which, I'm afraid, has so often been the fuel of unwise sexual desire through the centuries!)

2. *There was something seriously wrong with the marriage relationship*

This is the second reason which people often give for committing adultery – and it's not an unreasonable one. When a relationship is falling apart at the seams, it's all too easy to seek comfort in someone else's arms.

So infidelity is often the *result* of a troubled marriage, rather than its cause. However, there's very little doubt that adultery can also be the *cause* of enormous trouble in a marriage, as Sharon's rather unfortunate case history shows.

Like an awful lot of people whose letters turn up in my postbag, Sharon made the serious mistake of having a brief affair with one of her in-laws. (This isn't all that surprising, really – I'm afraid that people come into such close social contact with their in-laws that there's an alarming amount of opportunity for adultery with them.)

Anyway, one Christmas Sharon was left alone in the house with her brother-in-law, Frank, while everybody else went out for a walk. They'd both had rather more gin than was good for them, and they ended up in bed.

Under normal circumstances, they might have got away with a brief and silly episode of that sort, had it not been for the fact that two weeks later, Sharon realised she was pregnant.

This Yuletide conception was *not* greeted with great enthusiasm by Sharon's husband, since he had had a vasectomy, and knew perfectly well that the baby couldn't be his.

The end result of this shambles was that *two* marriages broke up, and a child was born with no legitimate father. I think you'll agree that it would have been rather wiser if Sharon and Frank had kept their clothes on that Christmas. . . .

On the other hand, I have to admit that some people do seem to get away with adultery *without* disastrous results, as Elaine's story shows.

Elaine's marriage had been getting rather dull and pedestrian, particularly as far as sex was concerned. She was a "career girl", and often away on business. And on one of these business trips, she spent a wild and passionate night with a handsome young customer.

The following morning, she reflected on the fact that sex had been very, very good with him. A less sensible woman might have been daft enough to decide that this meant that her relationship with her husband had no future. But Elaine was pretty bright, and she realised that *it was the romance and novelty of the situation which had made the previous night all so enjoyable.*

So, she went home with a resolve to put lots of novelty and romance into her relationship with her husband in future. That worked – and their sex life (and their marriage) never looked back.

Nonetheless, adultery is *not* to be recommended as a "cure" for marriage problems! It's a bit disquieting that recent surveys suggest that only about a quarter of all husbands say that they take adultery seriously.

With the AIDS figures increasing, they ought to take it very seriously indeed. . . .

Sex parties and orgies (and the rival Harley Street mobs)

In the 60s and 70s, sex parties and orgies were, I'm afraid, very common indeed in Britain. When I was working in a VD clinic, I sometimes saw the unfortunate results of all this. I particularly remember interviewing a not-particularly handsome bloke from Redhill and saying to him slightly incredulously: "You mean you did it with nineteen ladies in a single evening?" Needless to say, most of those ladies (and their gentlemen friends) had to be hauled in for treatment.

These orgies were certainly not confined to the seething fleshpots of Redhill and Dorking: for many years, staid old Harley Street itself – where you'd have thought the medical inhabitants would have known better – boasted two distinct orgy circuits.

One was run by a very, very distinguished British consultant, whose name is known throughout the medical world. I first began to get a bit suspicious of this chap in 1967, when he accidentally showed a bit of the wrong film at a university lecture: instead of a "clip" of a patient having treatment, we saw a naked lady advancing towards an enthusiastic gent. Naturally, the projector was hurriedly switched off!

I later met people who'd attended sex parties in his Harley Street consulting rooms. One woman told me that "they were quite good fun, but you had to put up with being screwed by some pretty awful looking people".

She painted a vivid picture of a room full of nubile women and handsome men – all mixed up with obese elderly doctors sporting huge operation scars and true-blue varicose veins. (*Not* quite my personal idea of romance, I'm afraid!) Lesbian "forfeits" and human "daisy chains" were a popular feature of these amazing gatherings.

Rather surprisingly, Dr. — managed to keep mention of his orgies out of the press until he (and many of his friends) became so geriatric that there wasn't much point in going on!

Less fortunate was the aptly-named Mr. Roger —, a very well-known London gynaecologist who master-minded a rival "sex party" set-up at his luxurious consulting rooms throughout a large part of the 1970s.

In the evenings, Mr. —'s premises echoed with the merry

shrieks of agreeable young actresses reaching climaxes (or perhaps pretending to?).

But very unluckily for Mr. —, the *News of the World* managed to infiltrate a couple of its reporters (one male, one female) into the parties. When their front page report landed on several million breakfast tables, the kissing had to stop. . . .

In the late 80s, orgies are still going on – but most participants are getting very worried indeed. The organisation which (I believe) is the biggest in this extremely dodgy field still advertises extensively, but in a discreet way.

But it's rumoured that its parties are far, far less adventurous than they once were – with people who used to embrace a dozen lovers in an evening now being reduced to

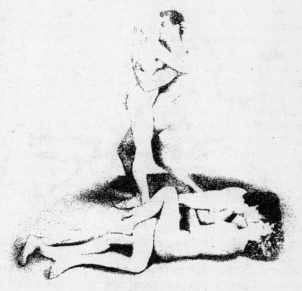

FIG. 12 Sex Parties

Sex parties – a good way to acquire chlamydia, thrush, and possibly even AIDS (not to mention p.u.o – pregnancy of unknown origin).

such safe but mundane activities as what I suppose might be termed "community masturbation".

Not altogether surprisingly, the Delvin Report found that only 4% of women said that they had been to an orgy.

But I was a bit disturbed by the fact that almost 20% of women said "I haven't tried it – but I might." I must say that to attend an orgy these days is *really* asking for trouble – unless, of course, you happen to be a reporter from the *News of the World*.

Threesomes (troilism)

Sexual "threesomes" are not as dodgy as orgies, because the risk of exposure to AIDS and other germs is obviously much less.

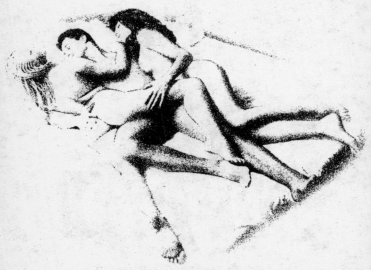

FIG. 13 Two Women, One Man

One type of "troilism": two women with one man – almost as difficult to do as it is to pronounce.

But as a form of "multi-partner sex", it clearly carries at least some dangers. Also, troilism – to give it its "posher" name – is (I believe) almost as difficult to do as it is to pronounce.

For instance, men tend to dream up amazing fantasies about having "three in a bed" sex with a lusty pair of women. But in practice, these "two women/one bloke" relationships do not (I'm told) tend to work out all that well – for the fairly obvious reason that it's not terribly easy for a

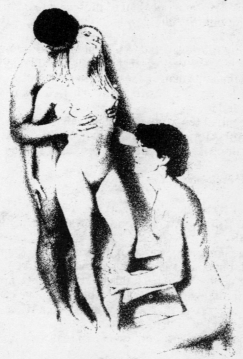

FIG. 14 Two Men, One Woman

The other type of troilism: two men with one woman – while this is the subject of many female fantasies, it's probably safer not to try it in real life.

male to satisfy two females. (Many men have great diffi-
culty in satisfying *one*!)

It is presumably a different matter if the two ladies have
any lesbian or bisexual inclinations – as in the recent
highly-publicised case in which Rambo, Mrs. Rambo and
her "girl friend" found their alleged bedtime activities
spread all over the newspapers.

But I'm not all that surprised that the Delvin Report
found that only 6% of respondents had tried "two women/
one man" sex – and only half of those had liked it.

What about the other kind of "threesomes" – two chaps
and a woman?

This might be expected to appeal more to women, many
of whom do have very erotic fantasies about being "taken"
by more than one man at a session (or even at the same time
– this is technically possible, though I certainly wouldn't
recommend it).

Three out of ten women told the Delvin Report that they
might try this form of troilism. But in practice, only 7% had
actually done it – and a third of those didn't enjoy it.

Open Marriages

Open marriages became almost par for the course in some
circles in Britain, America and elsewhere during the 1960s
and 1970s.

The general idea was that the man and woman were
married, but could sleep with whoever they liked.

I have no figures to back this up, but my own impression
(based on seeing quite a lot of "open marriage casualties"
in the surgery) is that a very high proportion of these
marriages ended in divorce.

Why? I think there were two main reasons:

★Jealousy;
★Falling in love.

1. *Jealousy*. Most human beings do have an amazingly
powerful jealous streak. So however civilised you may

68

think you are about letting your husband make love with somebody else, there's likely to come a time when you resent it – especially when he keeps on coming home from dear, sweet Cynthia's at 3a.m. (probably without enough energy left to make love to *you*).

In the case of husbands, this "open marriage jealousy" often takes the traditional male form of envy of the other bloke's equipment. Most men who attempt to run open marriages find it very difficult not to say to their wives: "Is Bill bigger than me?" or "Is Jim a better lover than me?"

If the wife unwisely answers "Yes" to either question, then the green-eyed monster is all too likely to start its work in poor old hubby's brain!

2. *Falling in love*. What people who go in for open marriages always forget is the very high possibility that either the husband or the wife will fall in love with one of the people they sleep with.

This happens so often as to be commonplace. I think this is because it's a fact that (particularly for women) sexual intercourse *isn't* just a triviality: it tends to have a strong "binding" effect on a relationship.

So it's very, very easy to fall in love with someone you've had sex with – specially if the sex was very good!

To be practical, open marriage should in my view (for what it's worth) now be a thing of the past. The risks of AIDS are really just far too great.

Wife Swapping

By the way, why does no-one ever call it "husband swapping?"

Although wife-swapping gets a lot of publicity – and is one of the commonest subjects of fantasy for both men and women – the fact is that only 3% of the married women who replied to the Delvin Report had actually tried it.

Many others said that they had found the idea a "turn-on", but only 8% were considering trying it out.

The whole idea has a bigger appeal (indeed a tremendous appeal) for many men. But men and women should understand that wife-swapping is emotionally risky, for exactly the same reasons that open marriages (see above) are emotionally risky.

Relationships which are just confined to two friendly couples should be free from the danger of AIDS and other late 20th century infections.

But *very* dodgy is the far more promiscuous type of wife-swapping practised by national "change-partners" organisations, which arrange for married couples to meet up with other like-minded pairs, "swap" for the night, and then move on.

The most up-market of these organisations is the one

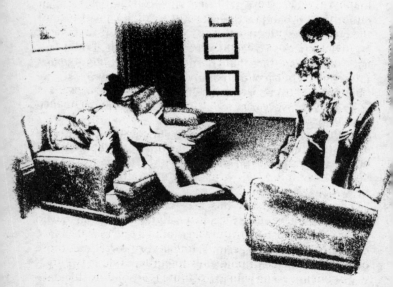

FIG. 15 Wife Swapping

Wife swapping: the lady on the right is already beginning to wonder if it was such a great idea. . . .

called "Nightshift", which is slightly unusual among wife-swapping clubs in having been the subject of a thoughtful profile in the *Guardian*!

Nightshift organises social events at which professional and other well-heeled couples can meet, listen to some agreeable music, take a glass of wine – and arrange to "swap" at a later date (Ascot and Glyndebourne permitting).

While this may all sound very attractive and "civilised", the sad fact is that as soon as one of Nightshift's thousands of members gets the AIDS virus, all Hell is going to be let loose, I'm afraid.

Prostitution

Finally a word about quite *the* most dangerous form of multi-partner sex (at least, for heterosexuals): prostitution.

The recent grim revelation by Deidre Sanders that *one in six* men has been with a prostitute fills me with dread.

Why? *Because prostitutes are rapidly becoming a major "reservoir" of the AIDS virus.*

This is mainly because so many of these poor girls are drug addicts, who work "on the game" in order to finance their craving for injected heroin.

In the course of a recent spectacular court case involving a prostitute, it was revealed that many of the girls are having sex with up to 800 men a month! If the men ask them if they have the AIDS virus, they naturally reply "No" – whatever the truth.

The implications of this are terrible. At the time of writing, a venereologist has just estimated that a man who goes with a British prostitute has about a one in 200 chance of catching the AIDS germ. Within a very short time, those odds must shorten dramatically to perhaps one in twenty.

To sum up: going with a prostitute is absolutely suicidal – even if you use a condom (which might easily split). You're probably coming into intimate contact with the secretions of the thirty or so men she's had in the last twenty-four hours. And you're also risking the viruses contributed by the thousands of men she may have had in the last year.

There are more sensible ways to commit suicide.

CHAPTER FIVE

Safe Sex Practices – And What The Delvin Report Revealed About Them

Yes, there are still nice (and safe) things you can do together • What the Delvin Report reveals about what men and women do in bed • Intercourse, and how often people do it • Simultaneous climax • Manual petting • Oral love play • Use of safe sex aids • Making love in varied positions • Making love on a water-bed • Turning each other on verbally • Making love in the bath or shower • Making love in Jacuzzis and swimming-pools, or in the sea • Making love in the kitchen • Making love in other unusual places • Erotic aids during sex • Love bites • Using massage, baby oil and other skin applications • Using wine, cream and other tasty items • Use of mirrors • Using video cameras • Use of fantasy • Summing up

Yes, there are still nice (and safe) things you can do together

Although we seem to be moving into a more puritanical era (forced into it by the AIDS crisis, I'm afraid), that doesn't mean that you can't go in for all sorts of jolly and exciting and slightly "naughty" activities together.

Indeed, doing such things is really a very valuable insurance against letting your marriage become dull.

And let me assure you that in the years when I worked in Family Planning Clinics, I saw all too many couples who'd done just that: they'd let the "sexual sparkle" go out of their love-lives, so that they'd grown bored and weary with sex. Very often, their marriages were in deep trouble as a result.

So read on: you'll find out in this chapter about what other people do – and you should certainly find some ideas that will help you to keep the zip and bounce in your relationship.

What the Delvin Report reveals about what men and women do in bed (and out of it)

The Delvin Report does reveal an astonishing variety of sexual practices among late 1980s women and their partners.

It shows that today's liberated ladies are willing to do all sorts of things in order to bring satisfaction and happiness to their partners – and (equally importantly) to themselves.

I think you may be surprised at how widespread certain love play techniques have become. In particular many people may be taken aback by the fact that oral love play (see below – literally) is now totally accepted by well over nine out of ten of all women – many of whom actually *need* it if they're going to get full satisfaction and achieve a climax.

Regrettably, many men don't realise this fact – and refuse to give their partners the one form of stimulation which they may need most if they're going to be fulfilled.

But before we launch into all that, let's just get our facts straight about what is, for nearly all of us, the nicest sex practice of all: intercourse, and how often people do it.

Intercourse, and how often people do it

Many people who returned the Delvin Report questionnaires made clear that for them good old-fashioned intercourse was the biggest "turn-on" of all.

Said Simone of Chelmsford: "I like all the way-out, sexy

74

things that my man thinks up to do to me. But my biggest thrill is to feel him driving deep, deep inside me, and knowing that he's just going to 'come', as far into my body as he can possibly go."

So intercourse is – fortunately for the human race – quite the most popular activity of all.

Now, how often do people do it? According to our findings, late 1980s woman is likely to make love 3.91 times a week on average.

This is quite a surprising figure, because it's well above the 2.4 times a week which has been quoted as the norm since Dr. Kinsey's surveys of nearly forty years ago.

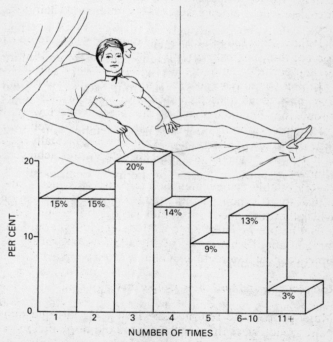

FIG. 16 How often women make love each week (Delvin Report); the average was 3.91 times a week.

I suspect that this apparent increase is a genuine reflection of the fact that these days, people are having more sex – simply because a) they're less inhibited; and b) effective contraception makes it so much safer.

One more fact about intercourse which may be of interest to you. We asked: "Would you expect your male partner to be able to make love to you more than once in the same evening?"

51% said "Yes"
42% said "No"
7% said "It varies"
1% said "Don't know"

Not altogether surprisingly, women aged under 20 had the highest expectation of their menfolk – with 73% of them expecting a man to be able to have intercourse more than once.

But even in the 40–59 age group, four out of ten women thought their men should be able to do it twice or more.

I have to say that these female expectations are more than a little optimistic! The truth is that very few men over the age of about 35 can make love more than once in an evening *except* with the aid of the most vigorous stimulation.

Only in men under twenty is repeated orgasm more or less the usual thing.

Simultaneous climax

Simultaneous orgasm is of course very agreeable – and the belief that it's "what should always happen" (fostered by so many romantic novelists) is still going strong.

In answer to the question "Do you think that trying to have a simultaneous climax is important?" almost a quarter of all women replied "Yes".

Among teenage girls (the under-20s), the proportion was even higher – at 36%.

In fact, I'm afraid that this is very unrealistic. You see, another question in the survey demonstrated (as we saw in Chapter Two) that simultaneous climaxes are really fairly uncommon. Most women actually *don't* experience simultaneous orgasm with their partners.

Only one woman in seven says that she "always" or "almost always" comes at the same time as her man.

Manual petting

I sometimes despair at the fact that so many women who've written to me say that their menfolk won't "pet" them manually – and that for this reason, they either can't reach orgasm, or else have to go in for a spot of DIY.

What on Earth is *wrong* with all you blokes out there? Surely you must have heard by now that virtually all women do need caressing by understanding fingers if they're going to be happy and fulfilled and orgasmic.

Nobody should consider himself a real man until he has at least mastered the two most basic manual caresses:

★The clitoral caress;
★The vaginal caress.

These are described in explicit – nay, graphic – detail, with full illustrations, in the companion books in this series *The Book of Love* and *How to Improve Your Sex Life*.

Nor should all you ladies out there neglect manual petting of your chaps. The woman who has developed a right hand skilled in this sort of caress is far more likely to keep her bloke happy and satisfied – and faithful. Again, full illustrated details of "How to handle a man" will be found in the two above-mentioned New English Library Paperbacks.

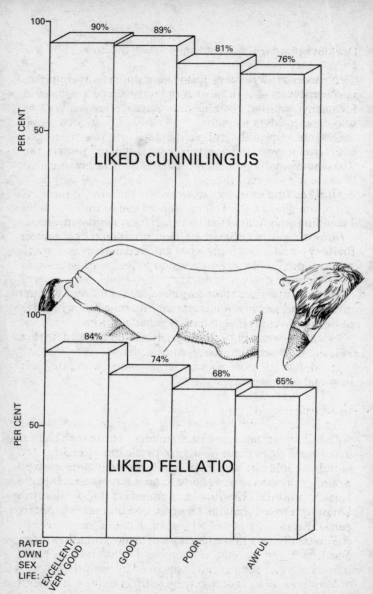

FIG. 17 The Delvin Report shows that oral love play is much more popular with women who rate their sex lives as "excellent" or "very good".

Oral love play

Some people still get very upset about this activity, but it's a very important part of most couples' sex lives today – and for many women, it's the only really effective way to achieve satisfaction.

Obviously, oral love play "divides" into two types: the man stimulating the woman ("cunnilingus"), and the woman stimulating the man ("fellatio" – possibly so called because it's more for fellers).

Oral sex (man stimulating woman). I'm sorry if puritans are offended, but the Delvin Report shows that this is an exceedingly popular activity – in fact, very nearly universal.

96% of women say they've been stimulated by a gent in this way – and the vast majority enjoyed it.

But there's still some opposition to it: 1% of ladies said they could *never* try it.

Oral sex (woman stimulating man). Slightly to my surprise, this is nearly as "acceptable" these days – with 93% of women having tried it, and 76% having enjoyed it.

But a substantial 11% of women disliked it, and a further 3% said they would never attempt it.

It's definitely most popular with women who rate their personal sex lives as "excellent".

Using safe sex aids

Again, this is a contentious subject. However, clinical experience does show that one particular sex aid – the vibrator – does help a very large number of women who wouldn't otherwise have done so to reach orgasm. Also, a battery-powered vibrator is perfectly *safe*. I wouldn't advise you to use a mains-powered one unless it's properly earthed.

Personally, I can't see much point in most other sex aids – and I've never encountered a patient who said that his or her sex life had been greatly improved by any other type.

However, there is certainly no harm in trying out sex aids

like clitoral stimulators and geisha balls if both of you like the idea.

In the Delvin Report, we asked women firstly about using a vibrator – and secondly about using other sex aids.

Using a Vibrator. Since the vibrator industry is now very big business indeed, perhaps it's not surprising that almost four out of ten women have used one. A further four out of ten say that they "might" try one.

Three-quarters of all those who've used one say they liked the experience.

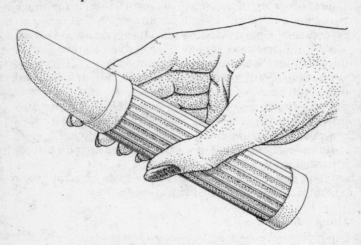

FIG. 18 A battery-powered vibrator.

But just over two out of ten women say they'd never use one.

Vibrator use (and satisfaction) are higher in older age groups, and very high in the "divorce/separated/widowed" group, which is not perhaps surprising.

Using other sex aids. In contrast to vibrators, these are scarcely known to most respondents. Only 8% of women have tried such aids – though over half of all women say they "might" try them.

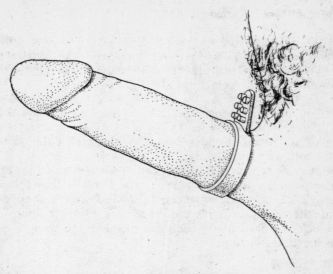

FIG. 19 Clitoral stimulator: the projection is supposed to stimulate the clitoris.

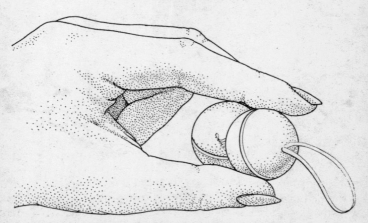

FIG. 20 Geisha balls. These are inserted into the vagina to give a vibratory "thrill"

Making love in varied positions

I still get letters in my postbag from people who've only ever made love in one position (invariably the "missionary" position, of course) and who wonder whether it might *just* be OK to try something else. . . .

Of course it is! As the vast majority of couples have found out for themselves, making love in all sorts of different positions helps to put a lot of new zest into a marriage. It also produces lots of exciting new sensations – for both women and men.

A wide range of differing positions is illustrated in the companion volume in this series *The Book of Love* (New English Library Paperbacks), but just to whet your appetite, here are four highly-erotic and very helpful positions – which are particularly useful in enabling the woman to achieve satisfaction.

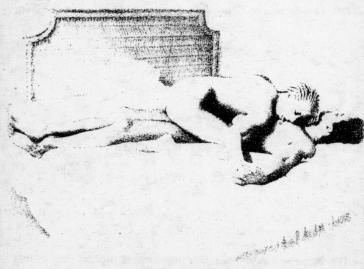

FIG. 21 The Mistress Position

1. The Mistress Position

Notice that the woman is on top of the man, playfully dominating him. In this position, she holds his arms down on the bed, and teases and stimulates his nipples with her tongue.

Although this position is a terrific turn-on for the gent, it's also very good for many a lady – because she feels "in charge", and also because (by pacing the way in which she rocks to and fro) she can precisely control the amount of stimulation she receives, and even decide exactly when she wants to climax.

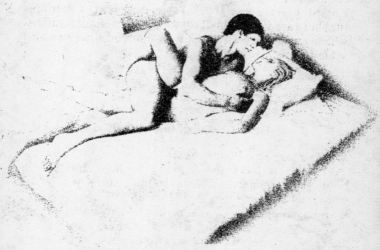

FIG. 22 The Tickle Position

2. The Tickle Position

In this cheerful "fun" position, the man is gently encircling the woman with his left arm.

He has her legs "trapped" with his right leg. (N.B. Of course, she's not *really* trapped, and could get free at any time if she wanted to.)

As you can see, he then uses his free right hand to tickle her armpits, neck and breasts as he starts to make love to her. As a rule, it's best to tickle for only a very short time, as not many women can stand this intense stimulation for more than a minute or so.

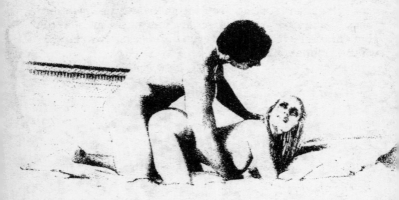

FIG. 23 The Doggy Fashion Position

3. The Doggy Fashion Position

No, this is NOT the name of an up-market canine boutique in Knightsbridge. From the picture, you can see exactly why the position is called by this name.

Some people aren't too keen on the idea of it – at least, until they've tried it. But it does produce a remarkable intensity of stimulation for many women, and it also has the great advantage that it leaves the man's right hand very free to reach round and caress her clitoris – if necessary, till she reaches orgasm.

This position is also particularly comfortable for ladies who're pregnant. And if you happen to be one of the substantial minority of women who have a "retroverted" ("tipped") womb, it's the best position for conceiving a baby.

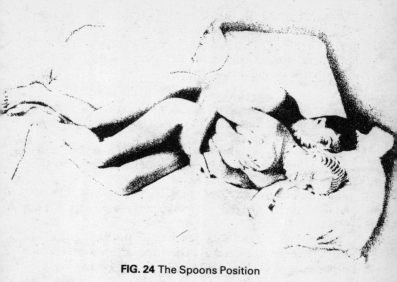

FIG. 24 The Spoons Position

4. *The Spoons*

So called because of the nice way your bodies curl round each other as the gent snuggles up to the lady's bottom.

This position has most of the advantages of the previous one, without being quite so "athletic".

Please don't laugh, but it's actually very useful for people with arthritis or rheumatism! In my agony uncle postbag, I get quite a few letters from couples who've reached the age when sex in the standard ("missionary") position is painful or awkward because of stiff joints.

Most of them have never heard of this position; yet for them it really is a very simple way to make love-making fun again – and to make it pain-free!

Making love on a water-bed

This can be a lot of fun, but in view of the high cost of water beds, perhaps it's not surprising that the Delvin Report found that only 6% of women have tried this! Two-thirds of them liked it.

3% of women said "I'd never try it". But a more aquatically-minded 89% said "I might".

Turning each other on verbally

This is what the Americans call "talking dirty" – *not* an expression I like myself, since there's nothing "dirty" about beautiful, loving sex.

So in the Delvin Report questionnaire, I asked women to say if they went in for "saying naughty things" to their partners in bed.

74% of ladies said "I've tried it", 56% said "I liked it" and 6% said "I disliked it". 8% said "I'd never try it", but 16% said "I might".

In general, women with "excellent" or "very good" sex lives were most likely to have tried and enjoyed this – which perhaps suggests that by and large it's good for you.

Making love in the bath or shower

I keep getting queries about this in my postbag, mainly from men whose wives want them to make love to them in the bath – but who are worried in case this will do the lady some harm by "pumping" water into her.

This certainly shouldn't happen: I recently spoke at a gynaecologists' dinner and asked the audience if they'd ever heard of a woman coming to harm through lovemaking in the bath. None of them had ever encountered such a case.

Anyway, in the Delvin Report questionnaire, I enquired about making love in the bath. 74% of women have tried this, and roughly two-thirds of them liked it. But about one in six didn't. (One woman – not unreasonably – mentioned "fear of drowning".)

4% of respondents said firmly "I'd never try making love in the bath", but a substantial 21% said, "I might try it".

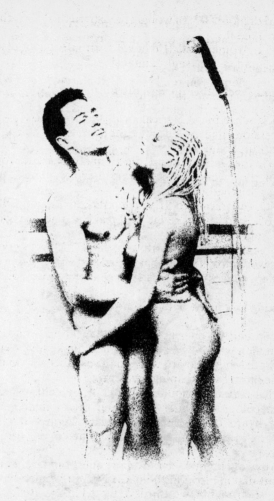

FIG. 25 Shower

Making love in the shower: many couples like the warmth and closeness of this – but be careful not to push the knob into the hot area of your control dial.

Bathroom love-making is commoner in the more mature age groups, and in married (and divorced) women.

It's rarer in the single, and among ladies who rate their sex lives as "awful".

If by chance you really are a bit alarmed by the idea of making love under the bathwater, an agreeable alternative is making it in the *shower* – which has all of the pleasant warmth, moisture and slipperiness of the bath, plus the erotic pounding of water in your ears – and all without any risk whatever of drowning! (Don't slip on the soap.)

Making love in Jacuzzis and swimming pools, or in the sea

I've recently received a couple of letters about babies which were conceived while swimming under water, so in the

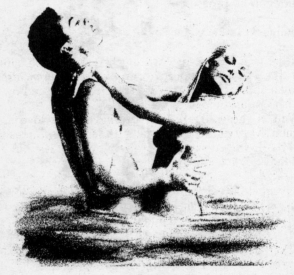

FIG. 26 Sea

Making love in the sea: the fact that a lot of couples enjoy having intercourse underwater has been confirmed by the in-depth research of the Delvin Report.

Delvin Report I was eager to find out just how common this kind of sub-aqua love-making really is.

Apparently, 23% of women have tried it, and the vast majority of those liked it.

9% of ladies said they'd never try this sort of thing. But a whopping 65% said they might.

Women in their 40s are the ones most likely to have made love in the sea.

Quite a number of respondents made the point that "making love in a Jacuzzi is fantastically sexy!" This is true: so is making love in any form of whirlpool or Scandinavian bath – particularly outdoors.

However, do bear in mind the recent case of the American women's volleyball team who went in a poorly-disinfected giant whirlpool bath together – and all got Legionnaire's disease.

Making love in the kitchen

Bearing in mind the recent French survey which showed that this was a common place for *les belles Françaises* to enjoy a spot of *pelotage*, I was interested to see how the British would compare.

Well, a surprising 49% of you have made love in the kitchen. Most of those enjoyed it, though 4% *disliked* it.

11% of women said they would never try it – but 37% said they might some time. Mind out for the wok.

P.S. Forgive my use of the Frog word *pelotage* above. In case you're not familiar with it, try looking it up in Harrap's French Dictionary; you'll find that it means:

(a) caressing or petting; and

(b) practising for tennis, or knocking the balls about. . . .

Making love in other exotic places

39% of women say they have tried making it in "other

exotic places", and scarcely any of them disliked the experience.

"Exotic places" which they specified in the Delvin Report included: on beaches; in cars; in trains (not British Rail, I hope); in aeroplanes; "in a loo at the ******* Club" (I trust this is meant to be a joke); and "in the cactus garden at Monte Carlo".

One intrepid lady made love "briefly and uncomfortably on a cloudy day at the top of the Empire State Building".

Using erotic aids during sex

In the Delvin Report questionnaire, I asked British women about their attitudes to certain quite exotic sexual practices – practices which might well shock some people, for instance:

★Looking at nude pictures during sex;
★Looking at erotic videos or films during sex;
★Bondage;
★Bottom smacking.

The results were surprising. Let's look at each activity in turn.

Looking at nude pictures during sex. One woman in three had tried this. We asked specifically about pictures of "nude men", "nude women", and "people having sex".

Contrary to what many males would believe, looking at photos of naked men is *not* very popular with women – only 14% liked it. In fact, looking at pictures of nude women during love-making is more popular – being liked by almost one woman in five.

A similar proportion liked pictures of couples making love. In general, older women are much more likely to look at such pictures than younger ones.

Looking at erotic videos/films during love-making. This kind of activity is of course highly controversial. But approximately a third of women have tried it (most of them liking it); a third say they might try it; and a third say they'd never try it.

Bondage (tying each other up). I have to admit that this is a practice which worries me – because it can be dangerous, and because it's sometimes used by blokes who are into violence against women.

But . . . one in five of all respondents have tried it, and just over half of those say they liked it.

However, nearly six women out of ten say "I'd never try it".

Bottom smacking. I'm not quite sure whose bottom is being smacked here! But three out of ten women say they've tried it – and half of those liked it.

For some reason which I can't work out, it seems to be more popular with ladies over the age of fifty. It's also more popular with those who rate their sex lives as "excellent". Some women said they could reach a climax through bottom patting.

Love bites

All doctors are aware that rather a large number of patients turn out to have love bites on their bodies when they take their clothes off.

So I was slightly surprised to find that only 72% of women say they've gone in for love bites – and that only half of these actually liked them. Love biting is decidedly more popular in the younger age groups.

Using massage, baby oil, and other skin applications

This is very popular nowadays. Two-thirds of all women have tried it – and nearly all of these liked it.

Very nearly everybody else said that they might give it a try.

Isn't that nice?

By the way, just plain ordinary *massage* is a great turn-on for most men and women. For both sexes, use a strong

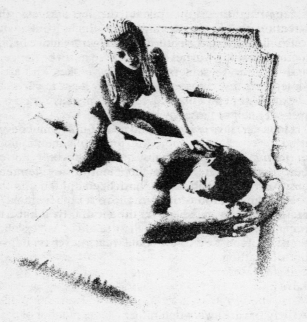

FIG. 27 Massage

Gentle, sensuous massage – for either sex, one of the best ways to relaxing and forgetting the cares of the day.

upward stroke on the muscles of the trunk and legs and arms, as shown in Figure 27.

If you're a woman massaging your feller (as we say in the advice columns), a good place to start is the area of the shoulders and the back of the neck.

Then move to the base of the spine, and make long, firm upward strokes towards his shoulder blades. Later, you can move to his arms, legs and tummy.

What about if you're a chap massaging your lady?

Well, one good way to begin is with that much-neglected part of the body, the toes. Stroke these one by one, kissing them betweenwhiles.

From her toes, progress up the legs, paying special attention to her calves and inner thighs (but *avoiding* touching her vulva or clitoris). Then gently move on to her tummy, shoulders – and breasts.

Applying, wine, cream and other tasty items to parts of the body as part of love play

This topic always seems to wind people up! Somebody once tried to report me to the GMC for simply mentioning the subject in one of my columns.

So I was surprised by the fact that most women reacted positively to the idea. Just over four out of ten said they'd tried it, and another four out of ten said they might. The vast majority of those who'd tried it said they liked using wine. *Santé*.

(But 16% of women said they would never try it.)

Using mirrors

What about making love in front of a mirror? Well, this activity is extremely popular.

Virtually half of all women who wrote in have tried it – and the vast majority of those enjoyed it.

Only 12% of respondents said "I'd never try it".

Note: you don't actually have to have the proverbial "mirror on the ceiling" to enjoy this one – though a mirror above the bed certainly provides some revealing experiences. But positioning your dressing-table mirror alongside the bed, or at the foot of it, will give you most interesting results.

Using video cameras

What about having a video camera on while you're making love?

Now that's a slightly different proposition from making love in front of a mirror, isn't it?

For a start, not all that many people have a video camera.

So I suppose we shouldn't be all that surprised that a minuscule 3% of respondents say they've done it.

And while a whopping 55% say "I'd never do it", a remarkable 40% say "I might".

Using fantasy

All authorities on sex therapy seem to agree that this is an excellent way of pepping things up in your marriage.

Just two words of warning, though:

★Never let fantasising get to become an obsession;
★Be very careful about deciding to turn your fantasies into reality.

You see, if a person keeps on and on thinking about some fantasy during love-making, it can get badly out of hand. For instance, the man who ALWAYS thinks about the woman next door while he's making love to his wife may well find that he ends up completely fixated on the lady next door – and unable to make love to his missus *unless* he thinks about the female neighbour.

Also, please heed that warning about "turning fantasy into reality". For instance, many women like to fantasise about running the risk of rape – or even being forced into sexual submission by a group of men. All very well perhaps as an erotic daydream – but the reality of rape is so ghastly that no-one who has been through it would ever want to run the risk of it again.

In the Delvin Report questionnaire, we asked women about two very common aspects of sexual fantasy. First: Fantasising about other men while you're making love. Sorry, gents – but virtually six out of ten women have done this.

Not altogether surprisingly, most of them enjoyed the experience.

However, one woman in four says she'd *never* do such a thing.

And then we asked about encouraging your man to fantasise about other women while making love. Not many women have this astoundingly generous trait! Only one woman in seven says that she's given this kind of encouragement in bed to her bloke. But most women who've done it say they've enjoyed the thrill.

On the other hand, nearly six in every ten women very prudently indicate that they wouldn't risk directing their partner's attention to other ladies' charms.

Summing up

So there are some interesting tips for spicing up your love-life, together with an indication of how commonly they're practised in Britain today.

In the next chapter, we'll be dealing with some rather more alarming revelations – about the frankly silly and dangerous things which far too many people do in the bedroom.

But let's conclude with a sort of "Top of the Pops" table of safe and enjoyable activities.

This batch of results seems to indicate that British women say that the commonest activities for spicing up their love-lives are:

1. Receiving oral love-play   (96%)
2. Giving oral love-play   (93%)
3. Saying naughty things in bed   (74%)
4. Making love in the bath   (74%)
5. Giving and receiving love bites   (72%)
6. Fantasising about other men while making
   love.   (57%)

Not for the first time, dear ladies, you amaze me with your sophistication and your honesty. Thank you all.

CHAPTER SIX

Dangerous Sex Practices – And Why They're Risky

What the Delvin Report revealed about dangerous sex practices ● Why do people do such barmy things? ● Spanking ● Whipping and sadism in the bedroom ● Having sex under the influence of drugs ● Rectal sexual games ● Heavy bondage ● Messing around with enemas ● "Water sports" ● Mutilation games and their horrendous risks ● Putting things where they shouldn't go

What the Delvin Report revealed about dangerous sex practices

Unfortunately, my survey does show that a surprisingly high proportion of British men and women do go in for bedroom practices that are risky or even downright dangerous – plus one or two which are actually illegal!

As you'll see from what follows in this chapter, the risky practices which I'm particularly concerned about in this AIDS era are the rectal ones.

If you shudder at that, and say to yourself that no heterosexual couple could *ever* go in for such games, I have to tell you frankly that you're wrong.

Because of the fact that the bottom is, I'm afraid, indisputably one of the erotic zones of the body, the truth is that not far off *half* of all women go in for love play games involving this area.

I'm not saying that this is morally wrong or anything like that: what I'm saying is that everybody should be well aware of the health risks. Read on.

Why do people do such barmy things?

Every time I mention any of these widespread but potentially dodgy practices in my advice columns, I get indignant letters from readers who say "Why would anybody possibly do *that* in the bedroom? My wife and I never would!"

Well, all I can say is that sex is a very, very powerful driving force, and that many couples are ever-eager to make it even more exciting and interesting by introducing new "variations" into their bedroom technique (which is quite OK, as long as the "variation" isn't dangerous).

In addition, it has to be admitted that there are an awful lot of people – mostly men – who are definitely rather "kinky" about certain sexual practices. Characteristically, these chaps don't really enjoy sex unless they're allowed to go in for their particular kink. (Indeed, they may not even be able to manage it at all unless they're doing whatever it is they particularly fancy.)

Why do people have these kinks?

Well, again and again it seems to be the case that a kinky person has some sort of fixation on *what happened in his early childhood.*

For instance, the rubber fetishist – who wants his wife to make love in a mackintosh – is probably harking back to the days of babyhood when he got some sexual pleasure, and perhaps some reassurance, from rolling round happily on that nice waterproof sheet. It's thought to be much the same with plastic and leather fetishists.

What about shoe fetishists? (These are the guys who want to clutch their girl friends' feet and kiss their high heels.)

They're thought to be subconsciously seeking the pleasure they got from being tickled by Mum's foot as they gurgled cheerfully on the nursery floor.

Of course, these are not dangerous "kinks". But some of the practices we'll come to in a moment, like flagellation (a love of being beaten) and heavy bondage (a love of being tied or strapped up) definitely could be.

Spanking

Spanking *within reason* is OK, and very large numbers of women appear to enjoy it – sometimes even reaching orgasm through being gently spanked.

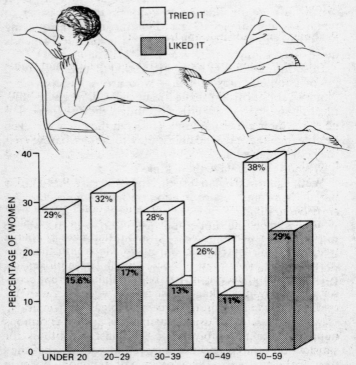

FIG. 28 Spanking (Delvin report). Overall, three out of ten women had tried spanking. Half of those liked it, but one third did not.

98

In the results of the Delvin Report, three out of ten women said they'd tried it – and half of those liked it.

It seems to be more popular with ladies over the age of 50. Also, it's more popular with those who rate their sex lives as "excellent".

But if bottom-smacking gets out of hand (so to speak), so that considerable pain is being inflicted, this really does suggest that something is wrong – and that someone may get physically damaged.

That risk is substantially greater if one of the participants wants to use implements, such as canes or whips (see below).

Whipping and sadism in the bedroom

What about when men start introducing whips, and wanting to lash their lady friends?

If you'll forgive me being subjective, this is an activity which worries me – mainly because I know what a lot of male sadists there are around.

I was faintly relieved to discover from the Delvin Report figures that only 5% of women have tried this – and only a minority of them liked it.

A whacking (sorry) 83% of women said "I'd never try it".

Seriously, beware of bedroom sadists: don't go out with them, and never marry them. Sometimes they kill people.

For completeness, I should add that there are of course vast numbers of men who introduce whips into the bedroom because *they* want to be whipped. These blokes are masochists, and once again it's thought that they're subconsciously "harking back" to some period when they were hit on the bottom as children and derived pleasure from it.

Masochists are not usually dangerous and an enormous number of them simply go to specialist prostitutes for satisfaction – often because they're not getting what they want from their wives. That's why half the phone boxes in our large cities are lined with sticky labels advertising the talents of "Miss Lash – Ex-Governess of Striking Appearance . . .".

Having sex under the influence of drugs

We only asked about love-making under the influence of *one* drug in the Delvin Report: "pot" (marijuana or ganja).

This is illegal in the UK, and we are not advising you to try it.

But 23% of women *have* tried having sex under its influence. And honesty compels me to report that almost eight out of ten of those say that they enjoyed it.

Since cannabis did not become popular in Britain till the 1960s, it's not surprising that using it for love play purposes seems to be confined almost entirely to women under 40.

Marijuana is not addictive and serious overdoses are rare – except when people are daft enough to use it in their cooking! Many authorities feel that it is actually less dangerous than alcohol. But the tell-tale smell could well bring the police to your door just as love-making is becoming agreeable. . . .

Far, far more serious are other drugs such as:

★Heroin;
★Amphetamines;
★LSD;
★Cocaine;
★"Crack" – the terrible new "instant-high" form of cocaine.

People are always using these to try and pep up their sex lives. This is quite crazy, as you're likely to end up impotent – or dead.

Nitrates ("snappers" or "poppers") are inhaled drugs which are sold openly *and legally* by sex shops. They are mainly used by homosexuals rather than heterosexuals – primarily for the curious "blast" they give to the circulation.

100

Having recently given evidence in a court case involving the sale of nitrates, I'd say that although these inhalants are said to be non-addictive, the risk of side-effects is sufficiently high to make their use unwise. Peter Sellers had been inhaling them during love play with Britt Ekland when he suffered a massive heart attack.

So in general, drugs and sex are NOT a good mix.

Rectal sexual games

In view of what we know about the mechanism of spreading of AIDS, I find the answers to the Delvin Report question on anal intercourse decidedly alarming.

Four out of ten women have tried it and roughly one quarter of these enjoyed the experience – but the majority disliked it.

I'm not greatly concerned about the fact that this activity – even between husband and wife – is illegal in England and Wales, and some other countries.

What *does* worry me is that the AIDS virus is spreading terrifyingly fast. So I'd strongly advise any woman who is letting a man do this to her to tell him to stop it – right away.

The only exception would be if a relationship is totally monogamous, when of course there should be no risk of introducing AIDS. But even then, a couple who are not careful about hygiene could easily transfer bowel germs from the woman's back passage to her vagina, and cause either a vaginal discharge or a urinary infection.

What about simple "bottom stroking"?

The caress of anal stimulation by hand (man stimulating woman) has become almost routine in some social circles. So maybe it's not surprising that 45% of women have been stimulated in this way. Rather more than half of them say "I liked it".

But there are some risks to this widespread activity. Maybe the 48% of women who say "I'd never try it" are being more sensible hygiene-wise. Anyway, a man who does it MUST wash his hand carefully afterwards – before putting it anywhere near his partner's vagina.

Again, the corresponding caress of anal stimulation by hand (woman stimulating man, technically known as *post-illionage*) is very widespread. Almost four in ten women say they've done it to their men – and most of these women enjoyed doing it. But 53% of respondents say "I'd never do it".

All I'd say is that if you do it, you MUST wash your hand afterwards. In particular, please don't get straight out of bed and start preparing an agreeable little post-coital supper without first scrubbing your finger nails. . . .

Heavy bondage

As we saw in Chapter Five, one in five of all women say they've tried some kind of bondage – and a little over half of them say they liked it.

Certainly, rather gentle and almost childish bondage games, like tying each other's wrists very loosely with a soft velvet ribbon, are quite harmless.

But "heavy bondage", in which the person is really *firmly* tied up (often so that he or she really cannot possibly get free), could be quite dangerous.

Particularly risky is the mind-blowingly stupid version of bondage in which the tied-up person is *gagged* by the other one. This can easily lead to suffocation, and deaths have occurred in this way. Don't try it.

Messing around with enemas

A study of prostitutes' advertising in central London reveals that an astonishing number of them are offering "enemas for gentlemen".

Yes, I'm afraid quite a few gents (and some women) do apparently get a sexual thrill out of being given an enema. Presumably this is partly because of the rectal stimulation involved.

Not all of these gentlemen are getting their enemas (or, if you're a Latin scholar *enemata*) from prostitutes. There's also an astounding trade in home enema gear.

Also, there are a number of up-market ladies – often nurses – who advertise their services in providing "colonic lavage". This is really just a sort of high-class enema, but the chap who pays for it can at least claim (and possibly feel) that he's doing it for the good of his health.

But is there anything wrong with this bizarre craze? Well, the one problem is that if an enema is given inexpertly – at too high a pressure or with too great a volume of water – it can burst the bowel!

Admittedly, such cases are rare. But if it happens, you really are in desperate trouble. . . .

"Water Sports"

The term "water sports" – so often seen in adverts placed by prostitutes in city centres – can mean enema administration (see above) *or* games involving passing urine.

Though you may find it a bit hard to believe, these urinary games seem to be quite popular, and people are forever writing in to certain magazines about them. (The link with early infancy seems fairly obvious here.)

But these watery antics could, depending on what you actually *do*, lead to the spread of viruses if one of you is infected with (say) AIDS or hepatitis.

In the Delvin Report, 9% of women said they'd gone in for urine games. Just over half of them did not like the experience. 81% of women said "I'd never try it".

Mutilation games and their horrendous risks

I am *not* going to describe sexual mutilation games, which became quite popular in California in the 60s and have to some extent spread to other Western countries.

Why? Because they're so obviously dangerous, and liable to lead to:

★Pain;
★Infection;
★Bleeding.

The very "mildest" form of this kind of thing is fitting body jewellery – putting gold rings or jewels in the nipples, penis or labia. Popping a diamond into one of the lips of the vulva received a great deal of publicity as a result of Sally Beauman's recent best-selling women's romantic novel, *Destiny*.

But even this is dangerous, and liable to introduce germs. Also, it could make love-making *very* uncomfortable.

Furthermore, you could easily lose your diamond. . . .

Putting things where they shouldn't go

In the days when I worked in gynaecology, I got fed up with removing objects that had been put into orifices which weren't intended for them, and which had got stuck.

These included:

★A jar of vanishing cream;
★An apple;
★An egg cup.

In one far more serious case, a wife suffered terrible damage when she let her husband penetrate her with a broom handle – what *stupidity*!

So clearly, you shouldn't insert objects where they aren't meant to go: this can cause big trouble.

To conclude this chapter on a less serious note, let me tell you about a young man who we saw in hospital whose "foreign body" was acquired as a result of a stag-night jape that went wrong.

His jolly – and very boozy – friends decided that they would "decorate" the nearly-unconscious bridegroom by pushing a flower into his male organ – the silly idiots! And when he attempted to remove it? Well, the fact that the leaves on the stem pointed upwards made it far more difficult to take out than it had been to put in. *So the head broke off in his hand.*

It took a general anaesthetic before we could get the stem out – and, yes, we *did* get him in shape for the wedding.

But the lesson is clear: don't stick foreign bodies in places which weren't designed for them!

CHAPTER SEVEN

The Facts About AIDS – And How It Could Affect You

Why it will affect every family in some way ● *Should we panic now, or later?* ● *What is AIDS, anyway?* ● *The symptoms* ● *The truth about how it's passed on* ● *Are there risks from social contact, food, crockery, swimming pools or communion cups?* ● *Who gets it?* ● *If you're a woman, could your husband/boy friends give it to you?* ● *If you're a man, could your wife/girl friends give it to you?* ● *How can you protect yourself?* ● *What risks are there in an affair?* ● *Where does AIDS come from?* ● *Where are you likeliest to catch it?* ● *How can you protect your children?* ● *Will Britain be wiped out by AIDS?* ● *Blood tests for AIDS.*

Why it will affect every family in some way

There's no point in trying to ignore AIDS, or attempting to convince yourself that it only affects homosexuals or drug addicts or Africans.

The number of cases of AIDS is eventually going to be so big that everyone is going to be touched by the tragedy of this disease in some way.

Unless you live in a very remote part of the world, it's a mathematical certainty that you or your family will come into contact with the people who have caught the HIV virus.

For I'm afraid it's quite inevitable that literally *millions* of British people are going to get the virus. As we'll see in a moment, it's almost impossible to forecast just how many of them will actually develop AIDS and die. But my bet is that the figure will be so high that most streets in the UK will have AIDS victims to mourn.

Should we panic now – or later?

Well, there's certainly no need for *women* to panic at the moment.

There is a widespread belief that British women are already in great danger. This is not true – *yet*. Of the 1300 or so cases of AIDS which have occurred in the UK, less than forty or so have been women.

Very few of these women caught AIDS simply through having "straight" sex with a man in this country. The following table shows how they caught the infection.

"STRAIGHT" SEX CONTACT IN BRITAIN	8	WOMEN
"STRAIGHT" SEX CONTACT ABROAD	10	WOMEN
INJECTED DRUG ABUSE	5	WOMEN
INFECTED BLOOD TRANSFUSION	8	WOMEN
BABIES FROM MOTHER	8	GIRLS
FROM NURSING INFECTED MAN AT HOME	1	WOMAN
FEMALE HAEMOPHILIAC	1	WOMAN

But . . . but . . . these figures are going to change dramatically. It's probable that *well over three thousand* British women are carrying the AIDS virus – but don't know it.

Sadly, many of those women will die over the next few years. And all of them are liable to infect the men they sleep with. So, it will go on – in a terrible human chain – unless we do something about it.

What about British *men*? The risk at the time of publication of this book is still surprisingly low *unless* you are:

★Homosexual;
★Bisexual;
★Haemophiliac;
★An injectable drug user.

But the risk for men, particularly those who sleep around, is increasing very fast indeed.

If you want to know your level of risk, then (whether you're male or female) you can do the self-assessment quiz in Chapter One.

What is AIDS, anyway?

AIDS is an infection caused by a virus, and viruses are germs which do not respond to treatment by penicillin and other antibiotics. This means there is virtually NO HOPE OF A CURE for many years to come. (It may be possible to develop a protective vaccine for healthy people – but that's going to take a long time, though one is on trial.)

The AIDS virus has a devilish ability to knock out your defences against infection, so that you won't die from AIDS but you will die from *chest or other infections* which a normal, healthy body could just shrug off.

"Kaposi's sarcoma" is a particularly unpleasant form of cancer which will affect around a fifth of AIDS victims. And recent research has shown that AIDS may often cause fatal *dementia* – particularly in children.

But it's important to realise that if you catch the HIV virus, it's by no means certain that you will develop AIDS.

We just don't know what proportion of HIV carriers will get the disease, but some have remained healthy several years after catching it. Others have developed relatively "minor" illnesses with fairly trivial symptoms such as fever and swollen glands.

The symptoms

We've just seen that AIDS does three things:

★It knocks out your resistance to infection – specially chest infection;

★It may give you an unusual form of skin cancer;

★It may cause dementia.

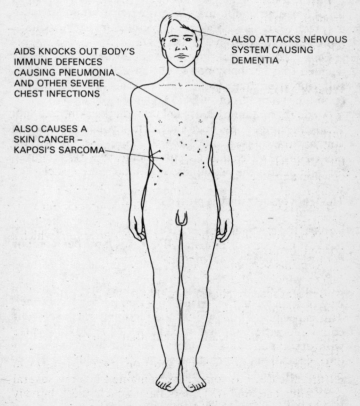

AIDS KNOCKS OUT BODY'S IMMUNE DEFENCES CAUSING PNEUMONIA AND OTHER SEVERE CHEST INFECTIONS

ALSO ATTACKS NERVOUS SYSTEM CAUSING DEMENTIA

ALSO CAUSES A SKIN CANCER – KAPOSI'S SARCOMA

FIG. 29 The main effects of AIDS.

So the main symptoms (which may come on anything from a few months to some years after exposure) are:

★Persistent cough which fails to clear up with routine treatment from your doctor;
★Odd-looking purplish swellings on the skin;
★Total loss of intellect – like premature senility.

Please don't "diagnose yourself" on the basis of this short list of the main symptoms. Unfortunately (but understandably) very large numbers of people are already deciding – quite wrongly – that they have AIDS.

One medically well-informed friend of mine recently decided that her baby boy might have it, because he was suffering from diarrhoea. (Diarrhoea is one of the less common symptoms of AIDS.) Of course, he didn't.

A cough, or a funny looking bump on the skin, or a spot of absent-mindedness do *not* mean that you have AIDS. If you have serious grounds for thinking you might have picked up the virus, then consult a doctor or AIDS counsellor, and discuss the possibility of a blood test (see below).

The truth about how it's passed on

Look at the graph alongside. You'll see that at the moment, the vast majority of British AIDS cases have been among homosexual or bisexual men.

Why?

Simply because rectal (or anal) sex is the most efficient way of transferring the virus from one person to another. This is because a) the wall of the rectum is very, very thin compared with the tough wall of the vagina; b) little cuts – with accompanying bleeding – happen again and again during rectal sex, which means that semen from an infected person can then enter the bloodstream.

Straight vaginal sex between heterosexual couples is not so likely to cause transfer of the AIDS virus. But it happens. A female carrier can transmit the virus via her vaginal

110

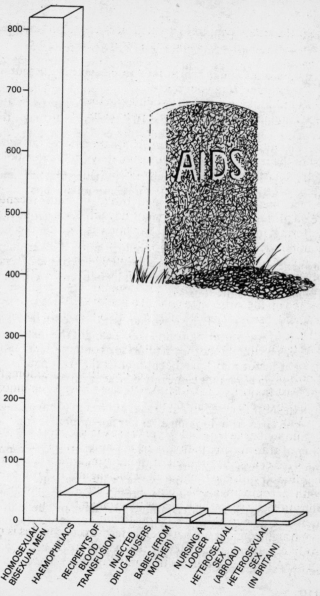

FIG. 30 Cases of AIDS in UK.

fluid – or a man can give to a woman in his semen. And in Africa this is already occurring *on a massive scale*.

This is really frightening – because if the African experience is repeated here, countless British men and women are going to become infected through vaginal intercourse.

The main way in which the virus spreads from the homosexual community to the straight one is through the AC/DC activities of bisexual blokes (see below) and through drug users sharing needles.

Are there risks from social contact, from nursing, or from food, crockery, swimming pools or communion cups?

"Social" transmission of AIDS – in other words, from ordinary social contact – appears to be not far off impossible. But contrary to what well-meaning Government propaganda has implied, there have been a couple of cases in which very close non-sexual contact between two people has led to transmission:

★In one case, a British woman who nursed her lodger (who was suffering from AIDS) caught the disease. It was claimed that they had no sex contact. An important factor may have been the fact that raw patches of skin on her hands came into contact with the poor guy's secretions.

★In another case, an American mother may have caught the virus from looking after her haemophiliac son.

However, the risk to nursing and medical personnel appears to be *very* slight. At the time of writing, no doctor has caught the disease from contact with a patient.

Also, about 2,000 health workers have accidentally "stuck" themselves with needles which have just been used on AIDS patients. Only one has become HIV positive.

Slightly more worryingly, several health workers who were accidentally splashed with "AIDS blood" have recently become positive.

112

What about other risks?

Food and drink and crockery. As far as we know, no-one has so far caught AIDS from food or drink prepared by someone with the virus. It seems most unlikely that buying a drink from a gay barman could give you AIDS!

Swimming pools. No cases are known to have resulted from swimming. It is hoped that the chlorine in swimming pools would kill the virus. Even if it didn't, it seems likely that swimming pool water would dilute the germs so much that it'd be very difficult for them to infect anyone.

Communion chalices. The risk of taking communion is reckoned by most experts to be small. But as the AIDS age advances (and as more clergymen die of it, I'm afraid) I think that a lot of churchgoers may go over to the alternative forms of communion – e.g. intinction – which doesn't involve sharing the chalice.

My forecast, for what it's worth, is that despite reassuring official propaganda, new ways of transmitting AIDS will be found as the years go by.

After all, among recent developments have been the discoveries that both artificial insemination (A.I.D.) and organ transplantation can transmit the virus.

The question of whether blood-sucking insects, such as mosquitoes, can pass on the germ is not yet resolved. Most experts say they *can't*, but personally I'll be happier when there's absolute proof of this.

Who gets it?

Figure 30 (above) makes the present situation clear.

The vast majority of British sufferers to date are *homosexual or bisexual men*. (Not homosexual or bisexual women, please note: lesbians very rarely get this disease.)

Then there are the poor old *haemophiliacs*. Between a third and a half of all the 5,000 haemophiliac boys and men in Britain now have the virus – thanks to the official bungling which let these completely innocent children and

113

adults be injected with a contaminated blood product from America.

Heterosexual victims of AIDS, who've caught it through straight sex are, as you can see, still small in number in Britain. But they're rapidly increasing in number.

Recipients of blood transfusions. This basically means people who were given infected blood some years back, before the AIDS threat was recognised.

All British blood is supposed to have been properly tested since late 1985. The same is not true of overseas transfusions, and in certain parts of the world, (notably Central Africa) you take your life in your hands if you have a transfusion, I'm afraid.

Injectable drug users. This category is increasing fast, particularly in Scotland. Unfortunately, many prostitutes are on injectable drugs. This makes them a major potential reservoir of AIDS – a pretty awful situation when you consider that, as we've seen, some of the girls sleep with hundreds of men a month.

If you're a woman, could your husband/boy friends give it to you?

Yes, I'm afraid so. This is especially likely if he is infected and you go in for rectal intercourse with him (according to our survey, this is practised by 40% of you). He can also give it to you through vaginal intercourse – and very possibly oral sex. The chances are less, though, if he uses a condom.

But remember, he can only give you the AIDS virus *if he's already got it himself*. You may think it impossible that your own husband or boy friend might have AIDS. But think again.

I thought that bisexual behaviour was very rare until I started to work in VD clinics in the early 70s. Overnight, I realised that it's actually very common indeed. Some women don't realise that vast numbers of apparently "straight" husbands and lovers are really bisexual. It has been estimated that around 15% of all men who go in for homosexual activity are married.

Another way in which your husband/lover could catch the virus (and so infect you) is through messing with injectable drugs and sharing needles.

Over the next few years, many husbands and boy friends are going to bring home the virus as a result of sleeping with other women – especially prostitutes.

If you're a man, could your wife/girl friends give it to you?

Yes, if she's acquired the virus elsewhere.

Vaginal intercourse is far from 100% effective at transmitting the virus from woman to man. But it happens, without any doubt at all.

So if your partner is promiscuous or is in one of the other high risk groups (e.g. a drug user) you must consider carefully whether you want your physical relationship to go on.

How can you protect yourself?

At the moment, the AIDS virus is principally a sexually transmitted disease the risk to yourself exists. (There are rumours that new variants of the virus may even be transmitted through breathing or coughing: I hope they're wrong.)

Firstly, make a mental resolution to watch your sexual behaviour very carefully over the next few years. Although the risk of heterosexual transmission was described as "remote" by the DHSS as late as December 1985, it's going to become very great during the 1990s. If you tend to "sleep around", be sensible and aim to stick to one partner over the next few years.

Secondly, make sure that your partner isn't a high-risk one. In particular, while I do feel very sorry for bisexual men, the fact remains that if I were a woman I would never have sex with one! The risk of AIDS is now much too great.

Thirdly, try to make sure your partner isn't promiscuous,

doesn't sleep with prostitutes, or go in for injectable drugs. Sadly, I have to add that a haemophiliac man would be a very high risk partner (unless he's been given a clean bill of health AIDS-wise).

Fourthly, if you stray from the paths of virtue with anyone other than your (hopefully) faithful partner, do use a sheath!

What risks are there in an affair?

If you have an affair with a heterosexual who is not a haemophiliac and not taking drugs, then your chances of catching AIDS are pretty remote, at the moment. But that's the late 1980s situation. By the 1990s a "one night stand" (particularly in the London area or in Edinburgh) will carry all the appeal of a game of Russian roulette.

Where does AIDS come from?

Figure 31 makes the likeliest theory clear. Admittedly, there's a fanciful theory that AIDS started in a CIA lab, but few experts believe that one. AIDS almost certainly started in Central and East Africa. That's where the disease is now on the rampage. (If you have to go there, do not have sex and avoid blood transfusions.) It probably spread to Haiti in the West Indies, which is a popular spot for American male gays. From there, it went to the gay "bathhouses" of New York and San Francisco – where unfortunately it was possible for a bloke to have sexual contact with fifty different men in a couple of hours. From America it was carried to gay clubs and brothels in Europe, especially Amsterdam, and to Australasia and the Far East.

Where are you likeliest to catch it?

Have a look at the map overleaf which shows the high-risk and low-risk areas of the UK. If you want to have an affair, you'd be well advised to have it in either Northern Ireland

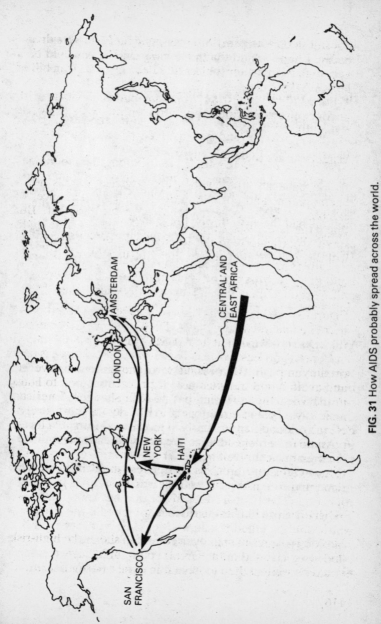

FIG. 31 How AIDS probably spread across the world.

or Wales at the moment! But alas *all of the British Isles* will become a high-risk area within a few years. Tragic, isn't it?

How can you protect your children?

Most children are likely to remain untouched by AIDS until they grow up and get involved in sexual activity – unless of course they're sexually abused.

The other main exceptions are a) young haemophiliac boys who've been tragically infected by contaminated blood products imported from America; and b) babies, who are in great danger of developing AIDS if their mothers had the virus during pregnancy.

If you are in any doubt that you may have contracted the virus, you should not get pregnant until you have been clinically tested and proved to be AIDS-free. Also bear in mind that the virus can be transmitted to babies in breast-milk – though that doesn't necessarily mean they'll get AIDS.

Will Britain be wiped out by AIDS?

Probably not. If the present terrifying increase in the number of AIDS cases continued, the entire population would be dead by 1997! But that shouldn't happen, because by the 1990s, the vast number of AIDS deaths must surely encourage people to live fairly monogamous lives. (In fact, in America the speed of increase is already dropping, presumably for this very reason.)

However the graph overleaf does show that at the moment the number of AIDS cases in Britain is really rocketing. The British Medical Journal has recently forecast that British AIDS deaths will soon equal the number who would be killed if a Jumbo jet crashed every month. And even more disturbingly, a secret Government report is alleged to claim that the number of AIDS cases could eventually exceed the number of hospital beds in the entire

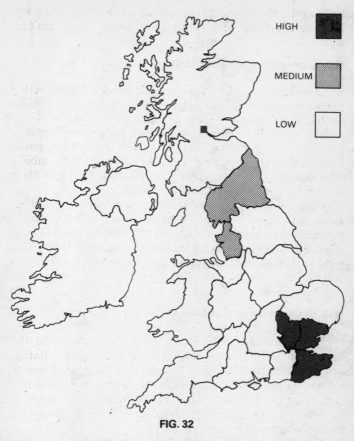

FIG. 32

country. That's probably why the DHSS keeps stressing that AIDS cases must if possible be nursed at home.

Blood tests for AIDS

During the next few years, as panic about AIDS increases, large numbers of people are going to want a blood test. But please bear these facts in mind:

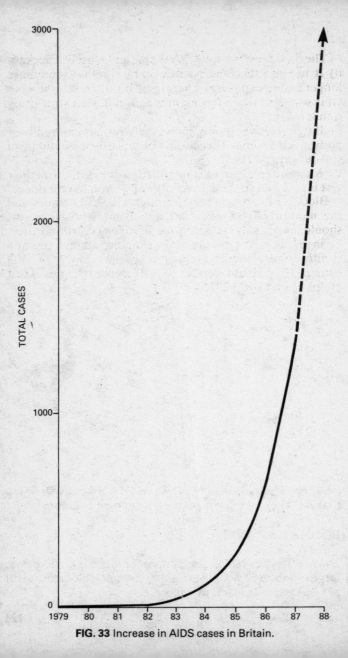

FIG. 33 Increase in AIDS cases in Britain.

a) The blood test is *not* 100% reliable and must be checked.
b) It may not become positive until months (sometimes longer) after exposure. Therefore, it only tells you what your situation was a few months ago, not what your situation is *today*.
c) If it is positive, it only shows the virus has entered your body at some time. This doesn't necessarily mean that you will develop AIDS.
d) Many people cannot cope with the knowledge that their test is positive, so think carefully before you have it done.

Blood tests are available through GPs, VD clinics and the new private clinics. Ideally, anyone who has a test should have highly specialised counselling before and after. So in my view, it's usually best to enquire about a test at a genito-urinary medical clinic ("special clinic" or VD clinic). If in doubt contact the Terrence Higgins Trust Helpline on 01-833 2971.

CHAPTER EIGHT

The Facts About Other Sex Dangers – And How To Avoid Them

Pelvic inflammatory disease (P.I.D.) ● *Cancer of the cervix* ● *Syphilis* ● *Gonorrhoea* ● *Thrush (Candida)* ● *Trichomonas* ● *Chlamydia and N.S.U.* ● *Unwanted pregnancy* ● *Abortion and its risks* ● *The emotional and marital risks of sleeping around*

Pelvic inflammatory disease (P.I.D.)

Unfortunately, women worldwide are suffering from an epidemic of pelvic inflammatory disease – P.I.D. for short. Yet most women have never heard of it!

What is it? It's an infection of the internal female organs, usually caused by germs which are introduced during sex.

For obvious reasons, it became far more common during the 60s, 70s and 80s – the period during which so many women started to go in for sex with a wide range of partners.

It causes one or more of the following symptoms:

★Pain;
★Discharge;
★Fever;
★Infertility.

122

Note that word "infertility" in particular, for I'm afraid that there are literally hundreds of thousands of British women who've had fertility problems because P.I.D. has blocked their tubes (just as in Figure 34).

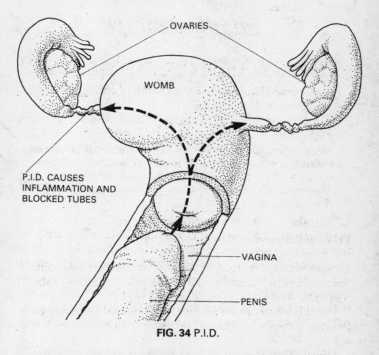

FIG. 34 P.I.D.

That's actually the main reason why so many people have had to try the "test tube baby technique" in order to overcome the problem of blockage of the tubes. Usually, the blockage has been caused by a germ introduced during some sexual encounter years before – just as in the case of Lucy (see Chapter One).

Germs which can do this to you include the bug that causes gonorrohea and (very commonly) a fairly recently discovered one called "chlamydia" (see below).

But if you want to protect yourself against the all too common condition of P.I.D., what do you do? Simply this:

★Don't sleep around;
★If you have more than one partner, consider the advantages of a protective "barrier" method (the cap or the condom);
★Think carefully before you decide to use an IUD (loop, coil); as explained in Chapter 10, these tend to be associated with pelvic infection, particularly if you have more than one lover.
★Go promptly to a "Special Clinic" (Genito-Urinary Medicine Clinic) if you have any symptoms of P.I.D.; fast and efficient treatment, with the right antibiotics, could save your fertility, and your health.

Herpes

I "introduced" herpes briefly in Chapter One. People get very frightened about it, which is understandable, as it's no fun to have. However, herpes is *not* as awful a condition as most people think. It's caused by a virus, and is very like the recurrent cold sores which you see on many people's lips. In this case, however, the recurrent cold sore is on the vulva, in the vagina, or on the cervix (or, in the man's case, on the penis). In women, the blisters may sometimes cause a total inability to pass urine.

Unfortunately, as with cold sores on the lip, herpes isn't yet curable, though drugs like acyclovir (Zovirax) do help. However, contrary to what so many people believe, the condition does often seem to burn itself out, so that the recurrences of painful blisters may eventually stop.

If you suspect you might have herpes, always seek specialist advice and treatment. You should not have sex until the doctor in charge of your case gives you the go-ahead.

If you become pregnant, you should tell your obstetrician that you have had herpes. In order to protect your baby, it may be necessary to deliver her/him by Caesarian.

Cancer of the cervix

I mentioned cancer of the cervix (the neck of the womb) briefly in Chapter One.

This condition is *partly* related to sex, because it seems to be commoner in women who:

★Have started sex early;
★Have had a lot of lovers.

Most people know those facts – because newspapers like to print sensational headlines saying things like: "SEX CANCER LINKED WITH TEENAGE ORGIES (SAYS TOP DOC)".

However, what most men and women don't know is that there seem to be *many* factors which cause this common cancer.

For instance, it's much commoner in women who:

★Have husbands in manual occupations;
★Live in Wales or the North of England;
★Are West Indian;
★Are smokers;
★Have had several children;
★Are over 35 (contrary to what most people imagine from reading headlines about "TEENAGE SEX CANCER HORROR", the peak incidence is in OAPs).

Symptoms. What are the symptoms? The chief ones are bleeding after sex, bleeding between periods, and sometimes deep pain provoked by sex.

But in fact, this disease can and should be stopped in its tracks *long before it can ever produce any symptoms (see below).*

Prevention. There's now considerable evidence that *barrier* methods of contraception (the cap or diaphragm, and the sheath) help protect a woman against cancer of the cervix.

Also, all doctors now agree that *all* adult women who have ever had sex should make sure they have regular 'Pap' smear tests.

What happens in a smear test is that the doctor uses a wooden spatula to scrape some cells off the cervix (the neck of the womb). She puts these on a glass slide, and sends it off to the laboratory for microscopic examination.

The point of the test is this: if there are any abnormal cells present, that gives very, very early warning of the disease – long before it causes any symptoms. And at that stage, it's nearly always curable by laser therapy or a small "cone biopsy" operation.

As I've said, cancer of the cervix does eventually produce symptoms – such as bleeding after intercourse and bleeding between periods. But by the time it produces these symptoms, it's awfully late in the day. It's far, far better to detect it ten or twenty years beforehand by the simple and – in most cases – painless technique of a smear test.

Syphilis

Fortunately, women (and most men) need scarcely worry about this disease at the moment – because (thank Heavens) it hasn't made a comeback during the years of the Permissive Society.

That's fortunate because, apart from AIDS, it's the most terrible of the venereal diseases. In Britain and many other countries, it's now very rare except in highly promiscuous male gays, so the chance of a heterosexual man or a woman getting it is remote. It is, however, more common in America (which is why they have pre-marriage blood tests for syphilis) and in a few more exotic parts of the world.

The chief symptom is a painless ulcer (raw patch) anywhere on the sex organs. You can see what I mean from Figure 35. This soon clears up and goes away – but the hideous disease persists internally. Blood tests (and tests on the ulcer, if it's still present) make the diagnosis clear. Treatment with adequate doses of penicillin is usually curative if given early.

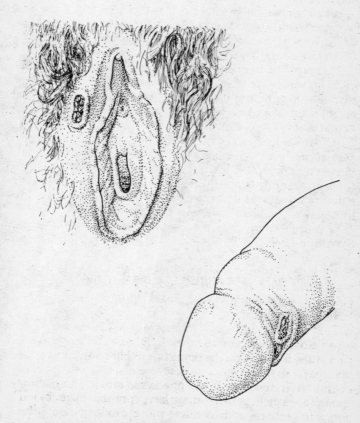

FIG. 35 Syphilis. It produces a painless "sore" in both women and men.

Gonorrhoea

Gonorrhoea (often known as "the clap") affects almost 60,000 people a year in Britain. It's worth knowing about, because it can badly affect your fertility, and your general health.

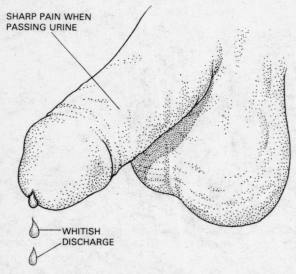

SHARP PAIN WHEN
PASSING URINE

WHITISH
DISCHARGE

FIG. 36 Symptoms of gonorrhoea and N.S.U. (urethritis) in men.

In men it causes:

★Pain on passing urine;
★A discharge from the penis (see Figure 36).

But what about women? Well, the tragic thing about gonorrhoea is that in most women it produces no symptoms. In some cases there may be an episode of pain, fever or vaginal discharge. But usually, what happens is that the woman makes love with somebody (perhaps someone she has a holiday romance with), becomes infected, but doesn't realise it.

For months or even years thereafter, the gonorrhoea germ may be damaging her health – and specifically the health of her pelvic organs. It may make her sterile, or give her P.I.D. (see above).

Fortunately, many women do have their cases diagnosed – because the infection is detected in their partner and he tells them that they need treatment. But the sad fact is that there's a very large number of women who are wandering around, quite unaware that they have gonorrhoea.

So, if you ever feel that you have 'taken a risk" (or if you suspect that your husband or boy friend has taken a risk by being unfaithful to you), consider the possibility of getting a full confidential check-up, preferably at a specialist genito-urinary clinic.

Once gonorrhoea has been successfully diagnosed, it can be treated – usually very successfully, if it's caught early enough. Treatment is usually with penicillin injections or capsules.

Thrush (Candida)

The dreaded thrush is by far the most common vaginal infection around today. It's a fungus which causes:

★Soreness of the vagina;
★Itching;
★Discharge, which is usually creamy white.

In men, thrush usually produces no symptoms, but some blokes become red and sore. However, the sex partner of a woman with thrush is very possibly carrying it. So both partners may need treatment with an anti-fungal cream.

If you think you have thrush, you should go to a doctor and have a vaginal swab taken, to confirm the diagnosis. The doctor will usually give you anti-fungus cream for your exterior surfaces, and anti-fungus pessaries (vaginal tablets) to clear things up inside.

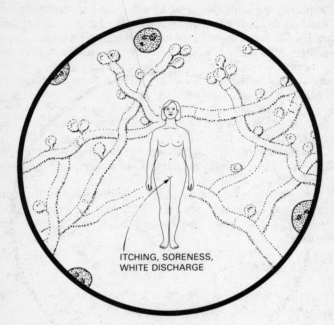

ITCHING, SORENESS,
WHITE DISCHARGE

FIG. 37 Thrush

Because the fungus loves warm, moist conditions, you should avoid tights, nylon pants, hot baths, and men – at least until the condition is cured!

In recurrent cases, Pill-users may have to consider switching to another contraceptive. If you're really desperate, try the remedy favoured by some feminist groups in the USA: apply yoghurt to the affected part!

Trichomonas

Say it "tri-ko-MOAN-ass." Trichomonas (also known as trichomonas vaginalis, or "TV" for short) is very common in women, in whom it produces a distressing vaginal discharge. You can see what it looks like under the microscope in Figure 38.

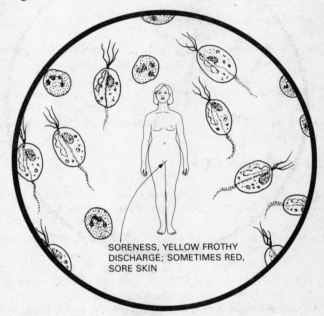

SORENESS, YELLOW FROTHY
DISCHARGE; SOMETIMES RED,
SORE SKIN

FIG. 38 Trichomonas

It's also *carried* by men, but it usually doesn't produce health problems in them.

Although there's some dispute about its method of transmission, it does seem to be passed on by sexual intercourse in nearly all cases. Catching it from a splash from a lavatory bowl, however, does seem to be a possibility.

Male partners of women with TV don't often get symptoms, though they might experience some pain in passing water. But they are *very* likely to be carriers – so they must be treated at the same time as the woman. Failure to treat the partner is the most common reason for the treatment of TV not to work. So make sure your husband/lover gets treated.

Symptoms of trichomonas are:

★Intensive vaginal soreness;
★Redness of the vagina and vulva;
★A discharge which is usually bubbly and yellow-green in colour.

Treatment – usually with an oral drug called metronidazole (Flagyl) – is, as a rule, highly effective.

But I repeat: BOTH of you must take it; otherwise you'll just get it back again.

Chlamydia (and N.S.U.)

This is a "new" infection, in the sense that it wasn't discovered all that long ago, and many people have never heard of it.

Yet millions of women world-wide have it, and in many cases it has affected their tubes and made them infertile by causing P.I.D. (see above). Regrettably, inexpensive tests for chlamydia aren't yet widely available (it doesn't show up on ordinary swabs). The result is that the condition often goes undiagnosed – and unfortunately, it's often treated with completely the wrong antibiotics.

Chlamydia should be suspected if a woman has persistent vaginal/pelvic pain, with or without a fever and a discharge. Salpingitis – that is, inflammation of the tubes (see Figure 39) – may be present. It's *vitally* important to get treatment with the right antibiotic – penicillin is useless, but erythromycin or tetracycline usually work.

In men, chlamydia often causes N.S.U. That's "non-specific urethritis" – by far the commonest form of sex

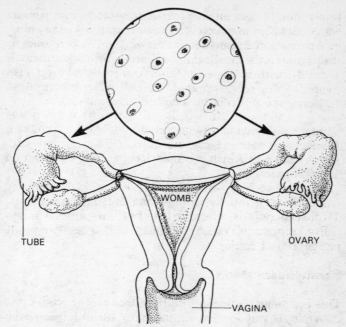

FIG. 39 Chlamydia: Today's new "epidemic" germ causes a variety of troubles including tube inflammation (salpingitis) and even arthritis.

infection in Britain today. Yet it's amazing that most members of the public have never heard of it!

Symptoms in men are similar to those of gonorrhoea (see Figure 36). Prompt treatment at a "special" clinic with the right antibiotics, plus careful follow-up and checking of female contacts, usually produces a cure.

Unwanted pregnancy

Though this sounds terribly obvious, unwanted pregnancy is one of THE big risks of unwise sex.

There are roughly 250,000 unwanted pregnancies a year

in Britain – which is completely crazy when you consider that almost 100% effective birth control is now available.

And the sad fact is that in a lot of these pregnancies, no one knows exactly who the father is. That's particularly common with what I call "the Benidorm babies" – the legion of tiny tots who are born each year as a result of frolics on the Costa Lotta the previous summer.

Again and again a British girl comes home from the summer holidays having cheerfully "bonked" with Juan, Manuel, Francesco, Pedro and José – not to mention Fred, Bill, Harry and Kevin (and probably Heinz, Helmut and Wolfgang too).

She then ends up with a sort of multi-national pregnancy – and not even any chance of getting an E.E.C. grant.

Honestly, it's a lot safer to avoid sleeping around and to use sensible contraceptive precautions. These are fully explained in Chapter 10.

Abortion and its risks

One pregnancy in five in Britain ends in being aborted.

While the physical risks of having an *early* abortion in an NHS hospital (or in a good private one) are very small indeed, they do exist.

For example, after a termination there's a slight chance of a womb or a tube infection, which could damage your fertility later on.

Repeated terminations are particularly likely to cause physical problems of this sort.

But in addition to the physical risks of abortion, there is the considerable danger of emotional harm. There's no doubt that both unwanted pregnancy and abortion can cause severe guilt and depression.

So the message really is pretty clear: if you have unprotected sex (and particularly if you sleep around), you are running a very high risk of ending up trying to get yourself a termination. Once again, it's a lot better to use the safe methods of contraception outlined in Chapter 10.

134

The emotional and marital risks of sleeping around

Finally, and without wishing to sound too puritanical, I have to say that as doctors, my colleagues and I do see a heck of a lot of the unfortunate emotional and marital consequences of sleeping around!

If your attitude to life is that you simply want to "screw anything that moves" (and that's a pretty common philosophy among a lot of men *and* women these days), you may get away with it for quite a while without doing anybody any harm. But in the long run, you'll almost certainly cause a good deal of emotional trauma to quite a few people – including possibly yourself. And you may well cause the break-up of good relationships – and even of marriages.

So, as we move out of the era of the Permissive Society and into the difficult years of the AIDS epoch, the fact is that for a variety of reasons – not least the emotional ones – it really is best to try to aim for "one-partner sex" if you possibly can.

Good luck.

CHAPTER NINE

Achieving Your Orgasm – And Achieving It Safely

What the Delvin Report revealed about orgasms ● Why you shouldn't let the search for orgasms dominate your sex life ● Secrets of easily orgasmic women ● What makes them "easy comers?" ● How they first reached orgasm ● What was first intercourse like for them? ● Are these women's partners something special? ● How they use fantasy in bed to reach a climax ● The importance of communication ● Where do they like being touched? ● Clitoral pleasure

What the Delvin Report revealed about orgasm

This chapter is basically about *women's* orgasms – because men don't usually have much trouble reaching one! (A few men can't climax; this condition is called "ejaculatory incompetence", and these days it can usually be successfully treated by a good sex therapist.)

In summary, what the Delvin Report showed about women's orgasms was this:

★The average age of first orgasms these days is fractionally below 20.
★On average, orgasm tends to occur *over two years* after you first start having intercourse: so there's nothing to worry about if you don't have a climax during the first year or two of love-making.

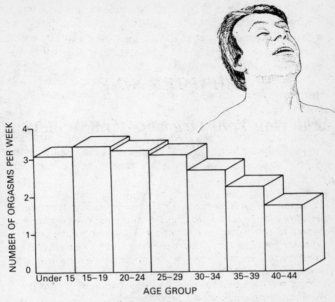

FIG. 40 Men's ability to reach orgasm at various ages.

★The average number of orgasms per week appears to be about 5½ (though many people are perfectly happy with far fewer).

★About 6% of women say they've never had an orgasm;

★Another 11% say they "don't often" have one;

★Only 13% of women *always* have an orgasm during intercourse.

★A very high proportion of female orgasms are achieved by petting (i.e. finger or mouth or tongue caressing) rather than actual intercourse.

★Simultaneous orgasm with your male partner is surprisingly rare: only one couple in seven achieve this "always" or "almost always".

★Almost six women out of ten now say they can have *multiple* orgasms if sufficiently stimulated – this figure

137

is far higher than it used to be back in the 50s, when only about 14% of women said they could do this.

★ 75% of women say that they masturbate till they reach an orgasm. Surprisingly, the figure is the same for *married* women.

Summing up, a lot more women are having a lot more orgasms these days.

But contrary to what you'd believe if you took romantic novels at face value ("As always, Lady Hermione attained the very zenith of her pleasure just as the Duke reached his own . . ."), women *don't* usually "come" simultaneously with their blokes.

In fact, most orgasms are probably obtained *outside*

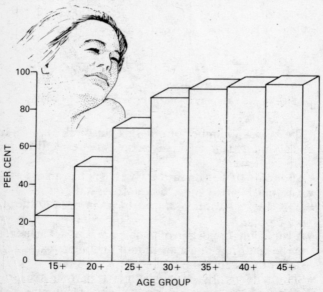

FIG. 41 Women's ability to "come" at various ages: note that the majority of younger women haven't yet reached orgasm. First orgasm tends to occur about 2 years after first intercourse on average.

intercourse – with a lot being achieved by the lady stimulating herself.

To say that all this is contrary to what most of us grew up believing about British married life is the understatement of the year. . . .

Why you shouldn't let the search for orgasms dominate your sex life

If you've read the above you'll realise that many people are very unrealistic in their search for "the perfect orgasm".

In fact, if you're enjoying your sex life (preferably with the man you love) and you don't feel frustrated or unhappy,

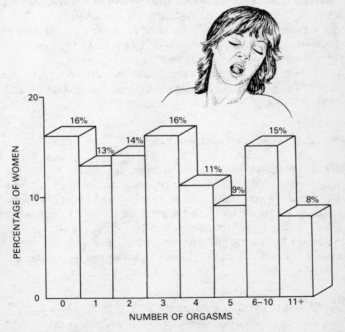

FIG. 42 Number of orgasms experienced by women each week (Delvin report).

then there's really no need to worry about exactly how many orgasms you achieve.

Incidentally, the Delvin Report figures suggest that you'll probably find it easier and easier to achieve orgasm as you get older. Many women seem to be still "improving" (if that's the right word) at the age of 50-plus.

What you *don't* want to do is to let the search for climaxes dominate your sex life. In particular, please don't make the mistake which so many women make, and move around from partner to partner, desperately seeking the one who will give them an orgasm.

For instance, my clinical experience has been that many highly promiscuous girls are not "bad" or "wicked" – they're just deeply insecure. They're worried about the fact that they don't seem to reach orgasm frequently (or at all), so they swan around going to bed with bloke after bloke, forever searching for the "magic" penis that they think will give them that elusive orgasm.

Orgasms are not the "be-all and end-all" of a relationship. However, it is of course very nice for you if you can learn to "come" easily.

Secrets of easily orgasmic women

Recent research in America by Marc and Judith Meshorer has shown that there is a substantial minority of women who've acquired the knack of reaching orgasm very, very easily – often by training themselves to do so. A few of these women can actually reach 100 climaxes in a single night – which certainly puts them on a par with the fabulously orgasmic Suzie of Leeds (who appears in Chapter Two)!

What makes them "easy comers"?

What makes a woman readily orgasmic? Research indicates that your upbringing and emotional development

140

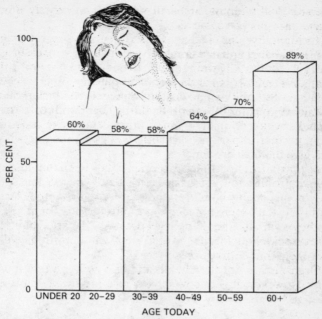

FIG. 43 Percentage of women who can reach multiple orgasms (Delvin report). Note how it increases with age!

play an important part in deciding whether you're going to be able to reach orgasm easily or not.

US studies have found that the following developmental factors are important in making women easily orgasmic:

★Having parents who "communicated positive attitudes about sexuality";
★Having parents who encouraged independence;
★Having a father who was "accessible" rather than "distant".

Astonishingly, a woman whose parents had an open attitude to sexuality, and who encouraged her independence, will become orgasmic *twice as quickly* as other women.

How they first reached orgasm

Many easily orgasmic women say that they first reached orgasm by employing what footballers call "the Diego Maradona method" – in other words, using your own right hand!

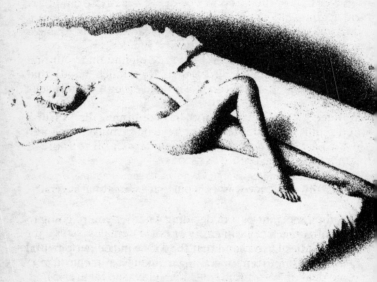

FIG. 44 Masturbation

The Delvin Report shows that the majority of women have done this – and that many of them have found it a useful way to relax and achieve orgasm for the first time.

Masturbation clearly helped them become familiar and comfortable with their own sexual feelings.

The work of sex clinics in this country and the USA has

confirmed this. If you're worried that you've never reached orgasm with a man, then just go to bed alone one quiet, relaxed afternoon and see if you can manage to make it *alone* through a spot of DIY.

What was first intercourse like for them?

You might assume that all ultra-orgasmic women had a really terrific time when they first experienced intercourse.

Not at all.

Over half of them report decidedly negative or indifferent feelings about first intercourse. In fact, only about a quarter of outstandingly orgasmic ladies seem to have actually *enjoyed* themselves the first time!

There's an obvious moral here: if you find that your first experience of sexual intercourse isn't much good, that doesn't mean that you can never develop into a really sexy person.

Indeed, the Delvin Report has confirmed the "thrills" and "spills" of first intercourse have been much over-rated in the past. It's actually *normal* to find it all a bit of a bore (if you'll forgive the phrase . . .).

Are easily orgasmic women's partners something special?

Yes they are!

Again and again, highly-orgasmic females stress the importance of having a loving and thoughtful partner *who wants to help you reach climaxes*, even if it means a very great deal of post-intercourse love play (see Figure 45).

I can't over-emphasise the importance of that last bit. Doctors keep finding that women who don't reach orgasm too easily will very often have husbands/boyfriends/lovers who couldn't ruddy well care less about assisting them to reach an orgasm!

For instance, I recently came across the case history of a highly attractive woman who'd only had four climaxes in ten years of marriage.

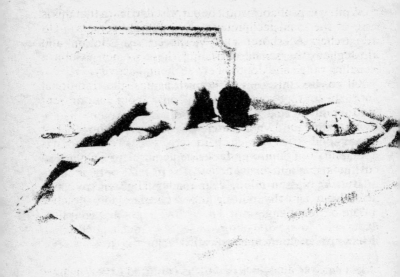

FIG. 45 Post-intercourse love play

It's very important for men to realise that when intercourse is finished, the woman may need a lot more love play with the lips or fingers to bring her to orgasm.

The reason?

Whenever she put her husband's finger on her clitoris, he immediately took it away – uttering the immortal words "I'm afraid that doesn't do anything for me, dear . . .".

The lesson is clear. If you want to have lots of orgasms, *get yourself a guy who likes making women "come"*.

After all, would you take your car to a garage where the mechanics didn't enjoy their work?

How they use fantasy in bed to reach a climax

The Delvin Report shows that nearly six out of ten women use fantasies of "other men" to turn themselves on while making love. (Sorry, gents, but there it is. . . .)

144

Well, you probably won't be surprised to learn that this is one of the main techniques used by "easy comers". US researchers Meshorer and Meshorer say "Before and throughout the sexual encounter these women exhibit a startling range and depth of erotic mental activity."

Of course, this goes very much against the traditional moral belief that you should think only about your present partner during sex.

Nonetheless, US research does clearly show that if there's one "trick" which characterises "easy comers", it is the ability to conjure up fantasies about being involved in all kinds of exotic sexual activity.

But do bear in mind, dear readers: fantasies are one thing, but actually putting those fantasies into practice might be very dangerous.

The importance of communication

Most "easy comers" say that they achieve what they achieve *by telling the man what they want him to do*.

That may sound obvious. But after all these years in the business, I can assure you that many (perhaps most) women are too embarrassed to tell their fellers to "rub there" or "kiss here". In their study of easily orgasmic women, Meshorer and Meshorer say that nearly every woman in their survey made the point that this kind of communication tops the list of basic tips of "How To Be More Orgasmic".

As one woman said: "I wasn't orgasmic for ten years – but only because I didn't tell lovers who were producing exciting sensations in me *to keep on going*."

Where do they like being touched?

Where do easily orgasmic women like being touched?

In both America and Britain, women who can climax easily say that they recommend getting their partners to stimulate all the "private bits" of their bodies:

- ★Ears
- ★Toes
- ★Buttocks
- ★Breasts
- ★Outer labia
- ★Inner labia
- ★Clitoris

Note: and when I say "stimulate", I do most definitely mean with the lips, as well as the hands. It has to be said that almost all "easy comers" find oral sex to be marvellously arousing.

And if this shocks you because you're opposed to oral sex, then remember that 96% of respondents to the Delvin Report said that they'd been on the receiving end of oral love play.

Clitoral pleasure

Finally, I can't emphasise strongly enough that nearly all ladies who can climax easily are quite uninhibited about wanting their clitorises stimulated.

About half of all easily-orgasmic women prefer direct stimulation of the clitoris – that is, rubbing or kissing the *end* of the clitoris, rather than the side or upper surface. The other half enjoy direct stimulation of the end of the clitoris, but they also like the sides and upper surface to be touched. Many of them also find that gentle rubbing with a vibrator is what helps them reach orgasm (see Figure 46).

But whichever way she wants her clitoris rubbed, the fact is that a multi-orgasmic woman is often so "successful" *simply because she has taught her partner to stimulate her clitoris in all kinds of different ways, frequently varying the tempo, the pressure and the precise location.*

Read and remember those words, gents: and you too may find that you suddenly have an easily-orgasmic lady on your hands. . . .

146

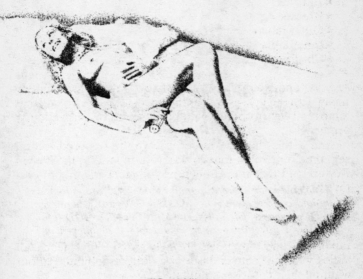

FIG. 46 Vibrator

Using a vibrator: the Delvin Report shows that about four out of 10 women have tried stimulating the clitoris with a vibrator, either from above or (as shown here) from below.

CHAPTER TEN

Safe (But Sexy) Ways To Use Contraception – Including How To Cope With Condoms

Which methods are most popular today? ● The condom: an up-and-coming method of safe sex ● The cap or diaphragm ● The sponge ● The Pill ● The Mini-Pill ● The IUD (loop, coil) and infection ● Spermicides and their alleged anti-AIDS activity ● Rhythm method ● Vasectomy ● Female sterilisation ● The Shot ● Effectiveness of the various methods ● A warning about abortion

Which methods are most popular today?

As we move into the AIDS era, it seems fairly obvious that people's attitudes to contraception are going to change.

For a start, it's suddenly become completely acceptable to talk about condoms! Until about 1987, you couldn't mention condoms on TV or radio or at dinner parties. Now they're on everybody's lips (so to speak).

But in fact the condom is still quite a way from regaining the position it once held as the most popular method of contraception in Britain.

The Delvin Report demonstrates this clearly. We asked women what method they were currently using, and here are the results:

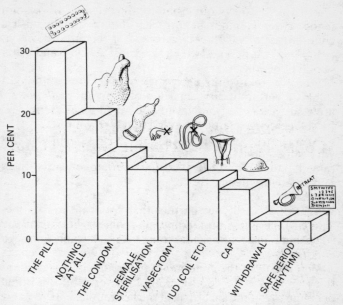

FIG. 47 Contraceptive survey: The Pill is still far and away the most popular method.

Note: some respondents were using more than one method – which was very wise of them, in my view.

Pill usage seems to be highest in the under-20 group – almost *two out of three* girls in this age group are taking it.

Male and female sterilisation were (not surprisingly) highest in the 40–49 age group. Indeed, four out of ten ladies in their 40s are relying on either male or female sterilisation for protection against pregnancy.

The condom – an up-and-coming method of safe sex

Although everybody seems to be talking about condoms, there's still a lot of resistance to using them.

But I have to say quite bluntly that anyone who is not living a totally monogamous life *should*, ideally, use a condom whenever they have sex. For this little device is really the best defence we have against AIDS – and other sexual infections too.

So if I were a young unmarried man or woman today, I think I'd certainly carry a packet of condoms *at all times* – after all, you never know who you might meet! Seriously, these inexpensive little sheaths could save your life.

Now, how do you use a condom? A lot of people aren't very sure about this. They make mistakes, get embarrassed, find they can't get it on – and perhaps end up with an unwanted pregnancy.

What you do is this:

First of all, tell your partner that you want to use one! There's no point in pretending, just come right out and say something like: "For both our sakes, I want to use a condom."

You must put the condom on *before* the penis goes into the vagina. It's no good making love for a bit, and then deciding to put the sheath on at the last moment. If you play things that way, you run some risk of pregnancy. You also throw away the anti-infection protection which the sheath gives you.

So, when you both feel you've had sufficient love play, take the condom out of its little foil packet. Be VERY careful not to tear it with your fingernails!

Don't blow it up to "test" it – it's already been very fully tested at the factory, thank you.

Just put it over the tip of the erect penis and roll it on. (If there's a little "teat" at the tip of it, then use your finger and thumb to press the air out of it *before* you roll it on.)

Now the "rolling on" process is what many men find difficult. Though not a lot of guys like to admit it, it's awfully easy to lose your erection at this moment! That's what a bloke usually means when he says "I can't get on with the condom".

It's very important that women should realise that the

moment of putting it on can be *very* difficult and embarrassing for a chap.

In fact, the most effective – as well as the sexiest – method of putting on the sheath is for the lady to do it for the gent, as shown in Figure 48.

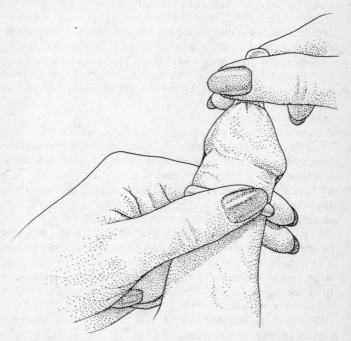

FIG. 48 The correct way to put a condom on your man. Squeeze the air from the teat before unrolling the sheath onto the penis.

If they do this as a natural part of their love play, with the woman gently stimulating the man with her fingers as she puts it on, then there should usually be no problems with loss of erection.

An alternative technique of putting on the condom is used by ladies of the night in Holland – as I discovered on a

151

recent trip to Amsterdam. (No, I *didn't* patronise the Red Light district; I learned about this from a Dutch venereologist.)

When they're faced with a punter who's nervous about using a condom (or who just plain *refuses* to use one) they resort to quite a subtle trick.

They offer the "john" a little preliminary oral sex. Before starting this, they conceal a French letter in the mouth. As the lips are closed over the penis, it's quite easy to slip the condom over it too!

In the dim light, the customer may never realise he's wearing a sheath until the encounter is all over. . . .

The cap or diaphragm

The cap or diaphragm probably does give a woman considerable protection against cancer of the cervix – because it forms a strong barrier between the tip of the penis and her cervix. (If you don't understand what cancer of the cervix is, please see Chapter Eight; and also Figure One, back in Chapter One.)

It may also give her *limited* protection against some sex infections. And although this hasn't been proved yet, I'd say – on commonsense grounds – that it'll provide at least some degree of barrier against the AIDS virus. However, this protection wouldn't be anything like as good as that offered by a condom.

In addition, the cap really is a jolly good method of contraception – about as effective as the sheath, though not quite as good as the Pill.

Now what is a cap? It's simply a rubber disc which the woman pops into her vagina (as you can see from Figure 49) in order to make a physical barrier that will keep the sperm from getting to the cervix.

It *must* be carefully chosen for "fit" in the first place by a doctor or nurse: because diaphragms (like women) come in many different sizes.

Also, it must be used with a chemical agent (a spermi-

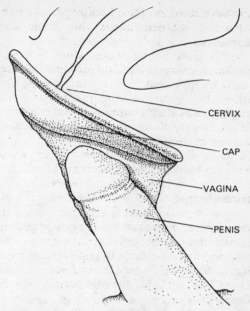

FIG. 49 The cap (diaphragm) in position during sex.

cidal cream or gel) which you put on it just before you want to use it. The spermicide lubricates the cap and makes it easier for you to put in; more importantly, it gives additional protection against pregnancy by stopping wily sperms from nipping round the edge!

Your diaphragm should be inserted no more than a couple of hours before you have sex, because the chemical agent loses its effect after a while. It should be left in for at least six hours after you've made love.

If you have intercourse a second time during those six hours (and if you do, you have my congratulations), you should "top up" the supply of spermicide by using an applicator to insert some more cream or spermicidal aerosol foam into your vagina.

153

Though the idea of having a cap inside you may seem "fiddly" or even distasteful at first, the fact is that many couples do find it an extremely useful method of contraception.

You may think that putting a cap in would take away the spontaneity of love-making. But there are two possible ways round this:

1. Young sexually-active women usually find it simplest to put the diaphragm in *every* night (say, when they clean their teeth); then it's ready in place if the couple decide to make love;

2. Other couples sometimes decide that the insertion of the diaphragm will become *a part of love play*. While this wouldn't be everybody's cup of tea, there are plenty of men who get a real turn-on from preparing the cap for the women they love – and then inserting it gently into the correct place in the vagina.

The sponge

This relatively new invention is shown in Figure 50. Marketed in Britain as the "Today Sponge", it's a simple use-once-and-throw-away barrier device which doesn't have to be fitted by a doctor. You just buy it over the counter at a pharmacy: there's no need to worry about size, as they're all the same.

The sponge is impregnated with a spermicide – which might just possibly have some *mild* anti-AIDS virus effect.

Most authorities think that the sponge is nowhere near as good as the cap or the sheath at preventing pregnancy. But it's certainly a heck of a lot better than nothing. Also, it's inexpensive, and quite pleasant and "feminine" to use: an important point for the fastidious woman.

Either the woman or the man can put it in at the very top of the vagina, right up by the cervix, as shown in the picture. Naturally, if the chap puts it in, this should be done as part of love play.

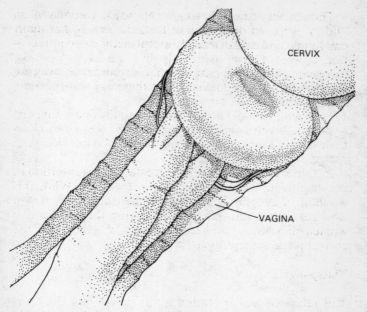

FIG. 50 The Today sponge being put into position with the finger tips.

In the morning, the sponge can be removed by pulling on the little loop of tape. It's then discarded.

Note: American research published just as this book was being completed suggests that the sponge has a high failure rate in women who've had children – possibly because their vaginas are wider.

The Pill

The Pill is far and away the most popular method among women who replied to the Delvin Report questionnaire. And indeed, though it's lost popularity just a little recently because of fears about cancer, the fact is that nearly a third of all sexually active women in Britain still take it.

The ordinary contraceptive Pill (as opposed to the Mini-Pill – see below) provides very nearly 100% reliability in protecting against unwanted pregnancy.

You take it for approximately three weeks out of every four (brands differ *very* slightly in this respect), and during the week off, you'll normally have a period. You can see this from the Pill chart in Figure 51.

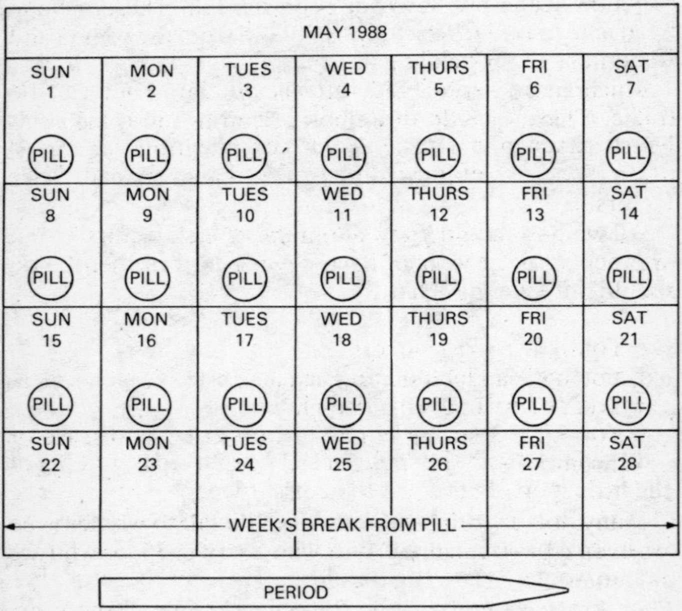

MAY 1988						
SUN 1	MON 2	TUES 3	WED 4	THURS 5	FRI 6	SAT 7
(PILL)	(PILL)	(PILL)	(PILL)	(PILL)	(PILL)	(PILL)
SUN 8	MON 9	TUES 10	WED 11	THURS 12	FRI 13	SAT 14
(PILL)	(PILL)	(PILL)	(PILL)	(PILL)	(PILL)	(PILL)
SUN 15	MON 16	TUES 17	WED 18	THURS 19	FRI 20	SAT 21
(PILL)	(PILL)	(PILL)	(PILL)	(PILL)	(PILL)	(PILL)
SUN 22	MON 23	TUES 24	WED 25	THURS 26	FRI 27	SAT 28
←———————— WEEK'S BREAK FROM PILL ————————→						

← PERIOD ————————→

FIG. 51 Taking the Pill, which must be done carefully – a recent survey found that 7 out of 10 women were doing it wrong!

What the Pill does during the three weeks that you take it is to *prevent you from ovulating* (producing an egg).

Good effects. There have been some reports suggesting that the Pill somehow helps to give a degree of protection against sexual infection – but I most certainly wouldn't bank on it!

More importantly, the Pill takes away period pain, makes periods shorter, lighter and generally more bearable, reduces the incidence of anaemia – and appears to help protect you against two serious cancers: cancer of the ovary, and cancer of the womb lining.

Bad effects. Minor – and usually passing – side-effects are common in the first few weeks on the Pill. These include headache, nausea, "spotting" of blood from the vagina and sometimes slight weight gain.

Much more serious side-effects are rare, but can be tragic. These include thrombosis (clotting) in a leg vein, heart attack and stroke. Such complications are most often seen in older women who have special "risk factors".

All women should know about these "risk factors" – but in practice, most women have never heard of them! You should not take the Pill if:

★You're a heavy smoker;
★You have high blood pressure;
★You're very badly overweight;
★You have a strong family history of heart disease or thrombosis.

Many doctors refuse to prescribe the Pill to women who are even *moderate* smokers, or who are over 35, or who are diabetic.

As knowledge about the Pill is increasing all the time, you must of course be advised by your doc or Family Planning Clinic as to what the current risks are – and whether you are suitable for it.

Don't hesitate to question the doctors about the question of *the Pill and cancer*. Although (as we've seen above) the Pill is now believed to protect you very considerably against two forms of female cancer, there are still doubts about whether it could increase the risk of:

★Cancer of the cervix;
★Cancer of the breast.

One or two *very* rare forms of tumour have also been linked with the Pill. So although it's an amazingly effective form of contraception, you should keep an eye on new developments – and don't hesitate to go back to the doctor or Family Planning Clinic if you're worried.

The Mini-Pill

This *isn't* a low-dose version of the Pill. It's a different product, which contains just one hormone – instead of the two hormones in the ordinary Pill.

This makes it slightly less effective. Also, it has to be taken *promptly* at more or less the same time every day: otherwise, you could get pregnant. You have to take it *every* day – without breaks.

The good thing about the Mini-Pill is that it appears at the moment to be much "milder" than the ordinary Pill.

So it's very useful for certain women who shouldn't really take the ordinary Pill: for instance, nursing mothers, or women who're well into their 40s.

The chief side-effect is irregular bleeding. To date, there is no known link with thrombosis or heart attacks. But of course, any drug could turn out to have alarming long-term effects after many years of use. Let's hope this doesn't happen with the Mini-Pill, which at present is a useful "mild" contraceptive for about 100,000 British women.

The IUD (loop, coil) and infection

You'll observe that nearly one woman in ten in our survey is using the IUD.

What is it?

Well, the letters stand for "Intra-Uterine Device". As you can see from Figure 52, it's an object smaller than your

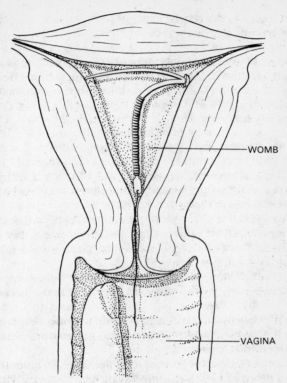

WOMB

VAGINA

FIG. 52 The IUD in position

little finger. It sits inside your uterus (womb), and prevents you getting pregnant.

It's pretty effective at this – though not quite as efficient as the Pill.

Older types of IUD were known as "the loop" or "the coil" because of their shape. Newer and smaller types are shaped like a "7" or a "T".

The IUD has to be put in by a doctor, ideally one who is *very* experienced in doing it, and not someone who has a bash occasionally!

She or he inserts it through your vagina, slipping it through the little hole in the middle of your cervix.

I must be frank and say that the insertion causes some pain – but most patients appear to regard it as far less traumatic than a visit to the dentist. On the other hand, a very small number of women do have quite a lot of pain and distress, and may feel quite faint.

Side-effects. The chief side-effects are heavy and prolonged periods and sometimes painful periods too. Also, the device very frequently comes out! (If this happens, don't panic: just don't have sex till it can be replaced.)

Rather more worrying is the question of *infection.* This area is still very controversial, but there does seem to be a lot of evidence that pelvic infections are commoner in women who have IUDs – particularly if they have quite a few sexual partners. The consequences of pelvic infection for your subsequent fertility can be pretty serious – please see "P.I.D." in Chapter Eight.

For this reason, doctors are now rather reluctant to fit IUDs into women who've never been pregnant. (If you've had a baby, insertion is much easier, and the risk of side-effects appears to be less.) Also, some IUDs have been withdrawn because their makers are terrified of being sued by infection victims.

Two other possible worries: if a pregnancy occurs while you're using an IUD (and this happens to about two out of every 100 women a year), it could well be *ectopic* – that is, in the tube.

Also, you should know that there's a small risk of an IUD going through the wall of the womb ("perforation"), particularly during insertion. The risk is reckoned to be very low – probably one in every 1,000 or 2,000 women – but you can see why I say that you should have your device inserted by a doctor who is putting them in all the time!

Spermicides – and their alleged anti-AIDS properties

Spermicides are, to be blunt, chemical sperm-killers. They

come in the form of creams, gels, pessaries, aerosols and little squares of film.

Despite what some manufacturers claim, they're no good by themselves, and should only be used as an extra protection with a cap, or a sheath or an IUD.

Recent reports have suggested that spermicides have some activity against the AIDS virus. That may be so – but I wouldn't depend on it if I were you! Still, every little helps.

One slight worry about spermicides: the American courts have recently started awarding huge damages to parents who have claimed that their children's congenital abnormalities were due to spermicides being in the vagina at the time of conception. The scientific evidence for this link is pretty unconvincing at the moment.

Rhythm method (and its variations)

Though well-meaning journalists keep ringing me up and assuring me that "everyone" is going over to natural family planning methods, you can see from our survey that variations of the rhythm method are still only being used by a tiny proportion of British women.

To be frank, this is mainly because the various types of rhythm method really aren't very effective. I'm sorry if saying that causes offence to anyone's religious feelings, but I think it's better to state the truth.

If you want to use the rhythm method (the "safe period") then you should use the best and most scientific variation of it available. *Don't* just rely on trying to calculate the safe period by juggling around the figures for your menstrual cycle.

At the present moment, I think that it's best to use a combination of the "temperature method" (in which you take your temperature daily, plot it on a graph, and work out when your ovulation time is), and the "Billings method". This is the technique developed by an Australian Catholic doctor, who pointed out that women's vaginal

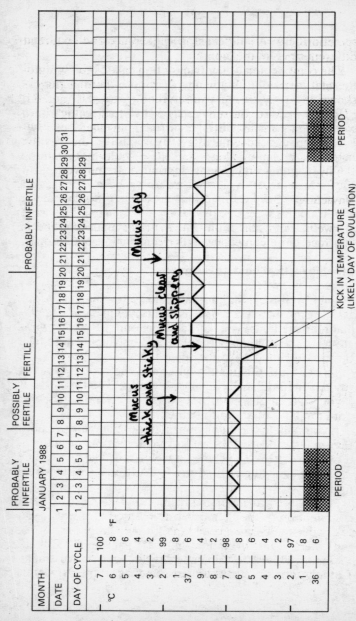

FIG. 53 Chart kept by a woman using the sympto-thermal variation of the rhythm method.

secretions are very different in appearance and texture at different times of the month.

The combination of the two is often called the "sympto-thermal method". One woman's sympto-thermal chart is shown in Figure 53. If you're going to try this method, *please* don't do-it-yourself: you need careful training from a clinic specialising in natural family planning methods.

Note: newer "chemical-test" variants of the rhythm method are coming along, and these could make natural family planning a much more attractive alternative.

Vasectomy

As we've seen, this is an increasingly popular method of contraception. Figure 54 makes clear what the operation is.

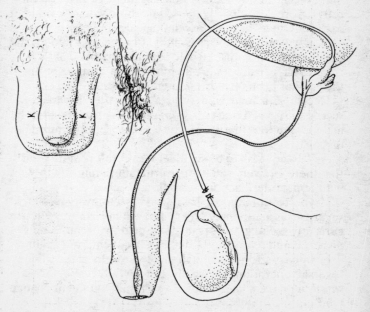

FIG. 54 Vasectomy

As you can see, the surgeon cuts through the two little pipes which carry sperm up from the balls to the penis.

This can be done either under local or under general anaesthetic. Either way, it's a very trivial operation.

Side-effects are usually trivial too, and mostly amount to no more than a little bruising and pain – or sometimes a little oozing of blood. (*Tip:* if it hurts after the op, get in the bath for an hour or so. This floats your testicles upwards, and so helps ease the ache.)

Very occasionally, a man suffers much more severe pain and swelling after the operation. This disaster happened to me (of course), and the full horrendous story will be revealed in my forthcoming memoirs. . . .

But to be serious, the operation will *not* make you sing soprano, or take away your virility, or remove your enjoyment of sex. However, all men should be counselled carefully beforehand – partly to exclude those who have hidden castration fears or other psychological problems.

You will still produce sex fluid after the op – and during the first few months, it will contain sperm. That's why couples have to use some other method of contraception till the guy has been tested and found to be safe.

Recently, a man who sired a baby after a vasectomy successfully sued the surgeon on the grounds that he hadn't been told that there was a small risk of failure with this op.

As *I* do not wish to be sued, let me therefore state clearly that there IS a very small long-term failure rate – as there is with female sterilisation (see below).

If you're thinking of having a vasectomy, you should regard it as permanent. Very large numbers of men are currently seeking "reversal" of vasectomy because they've divorced and re-married – and now want children again.

I can't say strongly enough that the results of the difficult reversal operation are really not awfully good. So you *shouldn't* have a vasectomy if you think you might change your mind.

A few men take out insurance by banking some sperm

with a private sperm bank. Obviously, this service is not available on the NHS, but the costs aren't high.

Female sterilisation

This op too is now fantastically popular, with one in nine of the respondents to the Delvin Report saying they've had it done.

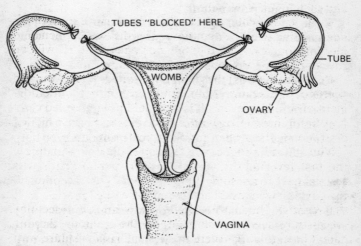

TUBES "BLOCKED" HERE

TUBE

WOMB

OVARY

VAGINA

FIG. 55 Sterilisation: the surgeon "blocks" the woman's tubes by tying, cutting or clipping them.

You can see what the operation involves from Figure 55. The surgeon "blocks" your two Fallopian tubes, sometimes by cutting through them, sometimes by putting clips on them, and occasionally by just tying them off.

The op can be done in three ways:

1. Through an incision in the lower part of the tummy (traditional sterilisation);

2. Through a cut in the upper part of the vagina (this is uncommon in Britain);

3. Using a telescope-like device inserted through a tiny

nick in the belly (this is called "laparoscopic sterilisation" and is used increasingly commonly in Britain today, because it's a much "milder" operation than the traditional one, with far faster discharge from hospital).

Here are just a few points to bear in mind if you're thinking of having a sterilisation:

★You will still have periods afterwards – contrary to what many people think†,
★The op does *not* give you the menopause (unless the surgeon decides to take your ovaries out for some reason);
★Sterilisation does have a small failure rate – so don't sue me if you get pregnant afterwards!
★Don't abandon birth control precaution till after the operation;
★Sterilisation is very difficult to reverse – particularly if the tubes have been cut. So be really sure that you both want it done.

The Shot

The Shot (or the Jab) is the controversial contraceptive injection. Only consider it if nothing else seems to suit you.

How does it work? Well, the woman has a jab in her buttock once every three months, and this stops her ovulating – giving her virtually 100% protection against pregnancy.

Very common side-effects include menstrual disruption, with either extremely heavy periods or no periods at all. Depression, headache and weight gain may occur.

The question of whether the Shot can cause cancer has not yet been fully resolved, but most experts think that it probably doesn't. However, you should take your doc's advice about this, and have regular cancer smear tests.

†*Note:* there is a theory that periods may be *heavier* after a sterilisation – but the evidence for this isn't yet convincing.

Unfortunately, the Shot has been given in the past by idiotic doctors who didn't tell women anything about possible side-effects – including one or two male, white doctors who (for curious sociological reasons) gave it to black women who were under general anaesthetic at the time, and therefore couldn't possibly give consent!

This sort of lunacy shouldn't be happening any more. In practice, the Shot is mainly given by female family planning doctors to women who are at their wits' end to find a suitable contraceptive – and who often beg the doctor to give the injection.

Effectiveness of the various methods

How effective are the various methods?

Well, here's a "league table" which shows my estimate of the number of pregnancies which would occur if 100 couples used each method for a year:

FEMALE STERILISATION	Nil
VASECTOMY	Nil
THE PILL	Nil
THE SHOT	Nil
THE IUD	2 or 3
THE MINI-PILL	2 or 3
THE CAP	3 or 4
THE SHEATH (CONDOM)	3 or 4
RHYTHM	5 to 15
THE SPONGE	5 to 20

From this you can see that all of the popular methods really are pretty safe. So accidental pregnancy these days should be quite uncommon – particularly if you use the various methods *sensibly* as outlined in this chapter.

A warning about abortion

I haven't given you a description of abortion – because of course it's not a method of contraception. But I should say that unfortunately, abortion is still very common: by my calculations, one in every five pregnancies in Britain is being terminated in this way.

If you become pregnant and feel that you should have a termination, please follow these rules:

1. Don't go to a back street abortionist: he or she may kill you.

2. Go to a doctor or pregnancy advisory service right away – abortion becomes more dangerous as pregnancy advances.

3. Always have adequate counselling – don't make your decision without the help of an experienced person who can discuss the pros and cons with you.

4. Don't let anybody "pressure" you into your decision: it's your body, and it's up to you to decide what to do.

5. If you decide to have a termination (and the doctors agree), please take great care to use adequate contraception afterwards – you don't want to have to come back for another one.

CHAPTER ELEVEN

Sex In The Nervous Nineties – And The Way Male/Female Relationships Are Changing

How sex is changing ● *The effects of the AIDS panic* ● *The puritan backlash* ● *Male/female relationships* ● *What will women expect of men in the 1990s?* ● *Safe sex*

How sex is changing

We're now at one of the great sexual "watersheds" of history, a time when people's bedroom behaviour is certain to change quite dramatically. In fact, I believe that the process has already begun.

What's happening? Well, let's look briefly at various different groups of people: gays; young singles; and the married.

Gay people. It's already quite clear from research done in Britain and the US that many gay *men* have altered their lifestyles drastically – and very wisely so too.

Although there is still a good deal of "cottaging" (that is, having a spot of quick sex with someone you pick up in a Gents' loo), there's now a strong tendency for gay males to try and establish more long-term monogamous relationships in the face of the AIDS threat.

There's no particular sign that gay *women* are altering their sexual lifestyles – but then lesbian women are prob-

169

ably at less risk of AIDS than any other sexually active group of people.

Young single people. At the time this book goes to press, many of the young single population of Europe and North America and Australasia seem to be "bonking" away like fury – as though trying to make the most of things before the AIDS menace finally strikes!

That must change. As soon as a few well-known heterosexual people start dying of AIDS, single men and women will surely get the message that indiscriminate and unprotected sex is absolutely crazy in the HIV era.

I personally forecast that when a famous woman film star dies of AIDS, the sales of condoms will sky-rocket. Furthermore, girls out on dates will start keeping their knickers on, for the first time in a quarter of a century. . . .

Married people. The Delvin Report figures have shown quite clearly that at the moment, adultery is absolutely epidemic in our society. In particular, women are being unfaithful far more than they were in the past.

Surely that too must change? In the Nervous Nineties, married people will have to realise that infidelity could well mean bringing home AIDS.

I am concerned that only just over one in four of those who took part in the Delvin Report say that the threat of AIDS is going to make them change their sexual behaviour – and that a mere 18% of teenagers are intending to be more careful.

But I believe those figures will change rapidly in the next year or two: as the gay community has already discovered, there's nothing like seeing a friend die to make you re-think your ideas about sex.

The effects of the AIDS panic

Unfortunately, the general alarm about the AIDS epidemic is already having some quite irrational results.

For instance, as I was completing this book I heard news of a sad case in which a woman had killed herself because

170

she was convinced that she'd caught AIDS. Tests showed that she had nothing wrong with her.

We've often seen this phenomenon in the past with other types of sexually transmitted disease: for example, every VD clinic has its quota of men and women who simply *cannot* be convinced that they do not have syphilis.

I would urge anybody who becomes terrified that they might have caught AIDS to seek professional help before jumping to conclusions (or off a building). In Britain, expert counselling is now available at any one of our 200-plus "Special Clinics" run by the NHS, and at some new private AIDS Clinics as well.

The general panic about AIDS is going to have some other odd effects too. I fully expect that people are going to become more "finicky" about hygiene, and to insist that standards of cleanliness and food-handling in restaurants, cafés and pubs are improved.

And though there's absolutely no evidence that AIDS can be transmitted through unhygienic food-handling, perhaps a little improvement in our national standards would be no bad thing at all!

The puritan backlash

I reckon that there can be no doubt that the tragedy which is just beginning to hit us will indeed cause a puritan backlash – primarily directed against people whose sexual morality or behaviour is relatively permissive or "liberal".

In the long run, this may well result in a reimposition of the constraints and censorship which existed in Western society up till the 1960s. If we're not careful, there may well be a return to the Dark Ages of sexual ignorance.

What's particularly worrying is that this backlash is very likely to include the persecution of gays.

Gays have had to fight very hard for their emancipation. It's not so long ago that male homosexuality was punishable by long terms in prison in most countries. I'm afraid that it seems very likely that the gay movement is going to lose

171

everything it has gained since then, as more and more people blame them for the spread of AIDS.

Already we're seeing ferociously "anti-gay" articles in some sections of the press. And as the AIDS epidemic builds up, it's almost inevitable that male gays will find themselves faced with job and social discrimination, and very possibly violence too. "Gay bashing" may well become a popular form of "revenge" for AIDS.

Rather bizarrely, there have already been reports of *female* gays being refused jobs "because of the risk of AIDS". This of course is complete lunacy, since lesbians are less likely than "straight" people to get AIDS.

Finally, in America we are already seeing yet another unpleasant aspect of the AIDS panic – discrimination against blacks, who are perceived by a lot of US citizens as being among "the causes" of AIDS.

The sooner we all realise that the HIV virus is a problem for the whole of the human race (not just for gays or blacks), the better.

Male/female relationships

Will male/female relationships change for the better in the next few years?

I sincerely hope so – though there's not much evidence of it so far!

We said to Delvin Report respondents: "Men are sometimes said to be more gentle and understanding these days. Do you think that where sex is concerned, the men you've come into contact with have changed very much in recent years?"

Less than four in ten women replied "Yes!"

Nor was there any great evidence that men were becoming more considerate *in bed*. For instance, we also asked the question *"Who decides when intercourse finishes – you or your man?"*

Well, I'm afraid that our results showed that the old male sexual selfishness is still winning here. In most relationships in the late 1980s, it's still the bloke who decides that love-making is over for the night.

51% of women said "My man decides".

Only 20% said "I decide".

Another 20% said "We both decide".

(And of course, 9% said "Don't know". After all, people do fall asleep. . . .)

I do hope that over the next few years we will at last see the emergence of the much-heralded "New Man" – the bloke who:

★Treats a woman as an equal – in and out of bed;
★Tries to share household tasks with her;
★Does his fair quota of "parenting" (like changing nappies . . .);
★Is considerate of her sexual needs;

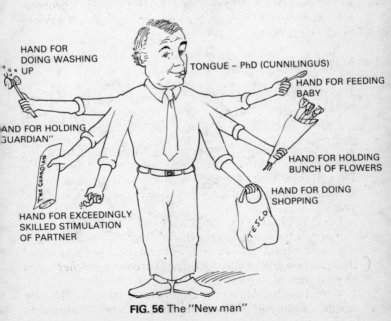

FIG. 56 The "New man"

173

★Attempts to make sure that SHE has an orgasm too (p'raps even *lots* of orgasms);
★Remembers that contraception is his responsibility as well as hers;
★Does his best not to give her VD – or AIDS.

What will women expect of men in the 1990s?

Well, the Delvin Report has thrown up some surprising (and occasionally bizarre) findings. Some are grim. For instance:

★The fact that so many women have been raped by men;
★The fact that so many recall being sexually abused as children – again, usually by men;
★The fact that a lot of women are still the victims of Stone Age sexual relationships, in which the man takes his pleasure with little or no thought for *her* sexual satisfaction.

But other findings are much more cheerful. For example, the fact that vast numbers of women appear to be enjoying their own sexuality with a gusto and a freedom that has probably never been equalled in human history.

Other discoveries of the Report are merely rather extra-ordinary: like the finding that *despite* what we "agony aunties" have been saying for years, a very substantial minority of women (one in three, in fact) do actually prefer a large penis!

So what does the Report suggest that women will expect of men in the 1990s? (No, sir: *not* larger phalluses. . . .)

Well, what comes through again and again from the thousands of personal letters which were sent in with the completed questionnaires is that:

★Women want more consideration in bed; and
★Women want more romance.

They *don't* want lots of "kinky" sex, as so many men

imagine: interest in this kind of thing was very low indeed. Cuddling, warmth and love were rated far higher than kinky gear and black leather!

As one woman said to me, "I just want to be loved and affirmed in bed as an equal."

That's the challenge of the 1990s, gentlemen. It's up to you.

Safe sex

Finally, whether we're men or women, let's remember that sex from now on has got to be *safe sex* – unless you want to wind up dead.

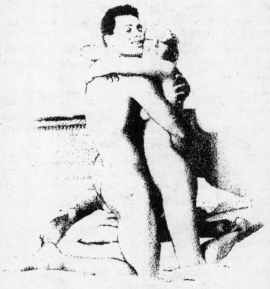

FIG. 57

The long erotic garden party of the 60s, 70s and 80s is over. From now on, it's got to be grown-up, responsible sex . . . or else.

FURTHER READING

Sexual Behavior in the Human Male, by Alfred Kinsey, Wardell Pomeroy & Clyde Martin; London: W. B. Saunders, 1948.

Sexual Behavior in the Human Female, by Alfred Kinsey, Wardell Pomeroy, Clyde Martin & Paul Gebhard; London: W. B. Saunders, 1953.

The Woman Report on Man, by Deidre Sanders; London: Sphere Books, 1987.

Ultimate Pleasure – How to Make Your Love Life Even Better, by Marc and Judith Meshorer; London: Ebury Press, 1987.

In Honour Bound, by Christine Webber; London: Century Hutchinson, 1987.